F
S

"Jaitara has birthed a profoundly awakening book on Sacred Sexuality that is rich in wisdom and practical insight.

She has done the deep work over decades within herself that allows the power of sexuality to take its rightful throne as a source of inspiration, healing, creativity, and ultimate pleasure.

If you've been hurt in relationships, tossed around with unclear boundaries, or haven't had the luck to find a mentor who knows the inside out of enlightened sex, then you have in your hands a priceless gift that will raise your sexual wisdom to great heights.

Devour The Four Sacred Laws of Sexual Enlightenment to help you realize your innermost desires and longings."

~ Satyen Raja; Founder of *WarriorSage Trainings*;
WarriorSage.com

"What an amazing, enlightening book! Jaitara really opened her heart and reached deep into mine in this book. I now feel like I know Jaitara personally and have been by her side through her journey.

Not many books have that feeling of a deep personal touch and trust. Jaitara shares a lot of valuable information in this book. I love how she takes you on a journey from animal spirits to orgasmic creation ceremony. I feel like this book is a gem that I was so lucky to find. Such an inspiration to connect deeper with spiritual guides, to invite divine source into the love making, to expand orgasmic energy and manifest sacred desires, whether with the partner or solo. I look forward to using practices and ceremonies from this book in my life.

And one more thing I think is worth mentioning - I'm very lucky to not have any sexual trauma but it looks like many women encountered some form of sexual abuse at some point in their life. This book is a miracle guide to healing."

~ Anastasia Barre; Virtual Assistant
and founder of VeryGoodVA.com

"VITAL INFORMATION FOR ALL INTERESTED in a truly spiritual life! This is a very beautiful and heartfelt sharing of Jaitara's life journey, and the lessons she learned along the way which she shares, to enable those who are looking for information to benefit from her experiences and wisdom in this process!

I am a seventy-eight year old widow of a sixty year incredible marriage. I have learned so much and am able to experience my life much more fully as a result of this information. The info in this book is valuable for all ages, I highly recommend it!"

~ Ginger Starr; Caregiver

"Gets straight to the heart of the matter. I absolutely loved the writing style. Jaitara makes you feel as though she is speaking directly to your heart. I love the power of her story telling and explanation of the practices she has used to have her breakthroughs. A very profound and moving book!"

~ Shayne Mrazek; Motivational Coach

"Sensual, authentic and liberating.

I have recommended this book to many of my friends. Jaitara is a beautiful person who has taught me many things including how to swallow fire. She has quite the life story that makes her qualified to write this healing book."

~ Katana Leigh Dufour; Artist; PaintInHawaii.com

Amy

Thank you for the blessing of your love, wisdom & beauty.

Love always
— Jaitara Jayde

"Jaitara is a pure expression of love and wisdom, who cares deeply for the expansion of love and joy in others."
~ **DON MIGUEL RUIZ**; Author of *The Four Agreements*

THE FOUR SACRED LAWS of *Sexual* ENLIGHTENMENT

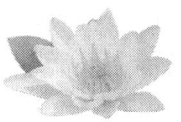

JAITARA JAYDE

Divine Sage Publishing

Copyright © 2019 by Jaitara Jayde

All rights reserved. No part of this book may be reproduced in any form or by any electronic or mechanical means, including information storage and retrieval systems, without written permission from the author and publisher, except for the use of brief quotations in a book review.

Cover design and cover art by Evelina Pentcheva
Sacred Sexual Enlightenment Wisdom Cards design and photography by Evelina Pentcheva; EvelinaPentcheva.com
Interior design by Jaitara Jayde: www.Jaitara.com

Foreword by Evelina Pentcheva
Editing: Janet Foster and Jaitara Jayde
Other books written by Jaitara: The Playful Partnership

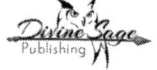

Divine Sage Publishing
1169 - 1685 H St.,
Blaine, WA 98230

If you are unable to order this book from your local bookseller, you may order directly from the publisher through the website:
www.DivineSagePublishing.com

Library of Congress Control Number: 2019938149

ISBN: 978-1-9995403-0-2

Printed on acid free paper in the United States

Limits of Liability and Disclaimer of Warranty:
The author and publisher shall not be liable for misuse of this material. This book is strictly for informational and entertainment purposes.

DEDICATION

*I dedicate this book to my mentors…
those in the physical realm, and to my nonphysical Divine Team,
who have enriched my journey with their guidance and love.*

*I dedicate this book to teens and young adults.
May you enter adulthood empowered by the
integrity, wisdom and beauty of Sacred Sexuality.*

APPRECIATION

To Spirit who surrounds me, I so appreciate you for always watching over me, guiding me as my Divine Team and serving me with your love. I adore how tangibly I consistently feel your presence and love. I love you back.

To my beautiful mother Marie, you were an unwavering presence of love throughout my life. You provided a shining light of acceptance and non-judgment that contributed to my healing path and my expansion as I grew to be the woman I am today. I miss you, Mom. Thank you for your love and the blessing of you.

My Soul Family of my dearest friends have given to me above and beyond, especially Howard Copeland for your incredible faith and unwavering support that allowed me the time and space to write this book and serve others.

Evelina Pentcheva, thank you for your sisterhood, love

and your extraordinary gifts of transformational photography and how you have lifted the essence of my brand, the message of my work, and the cover of this book to a magical realm. You are my soul sister. I adore the joy, love and wisdom you gift me with. I appreciate you deeply.

ANIBAL DIAZ AND JUNETH LOPEZ, thank you for the magic that you contribute through your images on the Sacred Sexual Enlightenment Wisdom Card Deck and in this book. The images of Divine Masculine presence and Divine Union are such a blessing and precious contribution.

DON MIGUEL RUIZ, I am touched by your love, humbled and honored by your support. Thank you the blessing and gift of you, for your mentorship and the wisdom of the Toltec Teachings and the richness and accountability they contribute to my life.

SATYEN RAJA, thank you for support, mentorship and love, and for how beautifully your teachings merge with mine.

JEFFREY ARMSTRONG thank you for teaching me the wisdom of the Vedic Teachings and how they enhance my message and my life.

TO ALL THE BELOVED SISTER FRIENDS in my life (you know who you are), you nourish and enrich my soul. It is always a joy to play, dance and share with you, and to celebrate life with you.

TO THE LOVERS who have blessed my life with your Divine Masculine essence and penetrated me on a heart and soul level, thank you for the beautiful reflection you have shown me. I hold each of you close to my heart for the love and connection we shared, and the wisdom gained.

FOREWORD

Two and a half years after I met Jaitara at an event her business card miraculously appeared on my desk.

A week later she called me...

The message she was sharing with the world was dear to my heart and I felt it was an honor to be of service through my artistic photography...

Although living hundreds of miles away, we've spent many days together at my home in California and at festivals.

Her spontaneous, innocent yet wise beyond measure nature is such a delight and a gift for my own spiritual journey. Her playfulness untouched by the years is inspiring and contagious.

Jaitara has a limitless ability to love unconditionally and nurture equally men and women. She is more than a friend. She is a sister, a mother, a guide, and to me a forever soul mate.

I perceive her as a channel of the Divine Mother.

In her veins boiling timeless wisdom...

In her spontaneity springing clear guidance.

Receive This book as a transmission beyond the words...

Let it become your pathless path to liberation of all illusion

Let it awaken infinite joy and absolute love in every cell of your sacred body...

and let it turn on within you the light of unbound pleasure that was always meant to be.

Thank you Jaitara, for giving birth to this magical creation.

~ Evelina Pentcheva; Artist, Transformational Photographer and Founder of *The Tantra of Presence*
TheTantraOfPresence.com

*Throughout this book you will experience cards from our co-creation, the oracle deck—*The Sacred Sexual Enlightenment Wisdom Cards*.

FOREWORD xvii

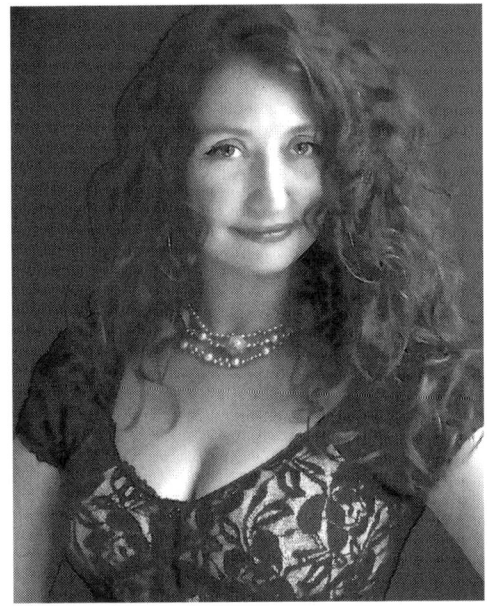

Evelina Pentcheva

ABOUT THE AUTHOR

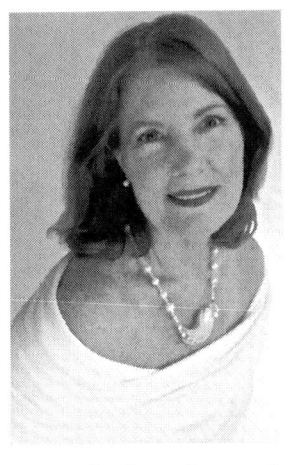

Jaitara supports lovers and creators, women and men, to live a life with more joy and pleasure... spiritually, sexually and emotionally, with or without a partner.

She does this through her wisdom teachings, and facilitation of *The Four Sacred Laws of Sexual Enlightenment* practices.

Jaitara facilitates healing through breath work and other techniques that clear emotional residue of past abuse and unhealthy relationships on a cellular level.

She guides women to be in the joy and power of their sensuality and pleasure.

She works privately with couples to deepen and enrich their intimate relationships.

She works with companies to teach men and women mindful communication for maintaining a harmonious and sexual harassment free workplace, as well as meditation to eliminate stress, and increase focus, calm and productivity.

Her story is powerful of how she healed her own wounds from adolescent exploitation, evolving into an inspiring role model of awakened feminine leadership, wisdom, and compassion.

Now in her 60's she still loves to dance like no one is watching. She serves others with the love and tenderness of a mother, the wisdom of an elder, and with youthful vitality and playfulness.

Jaitara is a certified Holistic Rebirther, Reiki Master Teacher, Cuddle Party Facilitator and personal development coach. She is a master facilitator of healing, breath, meditation, transformational dance, playful expression, and is an ordained Priestess.

The name Jaitara means, "Hail the Mother of Liberation." Her name came to her in 2009, upon waking one morning, following a prayer from the night before to receive her Spirit name. This name is a perfect balance in numerology with Jaitara's birthdate.

She was born in Halifax, Nova Scotia, moved to Toronto in 1983, then to Vancouver BC in 2001. Her co-creative partner Evelina Pentcheva, who designed the cover of this book and co-created the *Sacred Sexual Enlightenment Wisdom Card* deck with Jaitara, lives in Southern California, where Jaitara travels often, to visit Evelina and the rest of her California soul family.

Jaitara is a full member of ACTRA, the Canadian Actor's Union for film and TV and still dabbles in the business from time to time.

Her online and live events guide her participants on deep transformational journeys of healing and awakening, spiced with playfulness, through connection, celebration and dance.

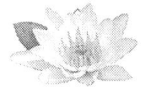

"Jaitara, the space you are able to hold in your sessions is very unique—and I have tried A LOT throughout my life. The Goddess Mother Embodied." ~ Eva Charlotte; Founder of R.I.S.E. In Love™, and Global Peacemakers™

CONTENTS

PART 1
THE JOURNEY TO DISCOVERY
Prelude to The Four Sacred Laws

1. The Day Of The Grackle	3
2. Bear Medicine	15
3. History And Herstory	31
4. Sexual Evolution	49

PART 2
THE FOUR SACRED LAWS OF
SEXUAL ENLIGHTENMENT

5. The Gift	61
- The Gift of Life	62
- The Body Temple	63
- Multiple Dimensions of the Gift	68
- Dance of Masculine and Feminine	74
- The Five Elements of Sexual Expression	90
- Summary	98
- Applying the 1st Sacred Law to the Work Place	99
6. Forgiveness	101
- The Gift of Forgiveness	101
- For Health	104
- Marriage and Other Intimate Relationships	107
- Family Legacy	109
- Sexual Abuse	114
- Forgiveness of Self	116
- Energy in Motion	118
- Forgiveness Process	119
- Summary	127
- Applying the 2nd Sacred Law to the Work Place	127

7. Responsibility — 129
   - Responsibility to Truth — 129
   - Responsibility to Healing — 131
   - Responsibility of Communication — 131
   - Responsibility of Consent — 151
   - Responsibility of Discernment — 154
   - Responsibility of Lifestyle Compatibility — 156
   - Responsibility of Body Awareness — 160
   - Responsibility of Reflection — 168
   - Responsibility of Acceptance — 171
   - Responsibility of Power — 173
   - Summary — 179
   - Applying the 3rd Sacred Law to the Work Place — 179

8. The Invitation — 181
   - Sex, God and You — 182
   - Miraculous Cycle and Brilliance of Breath — 187
   - Light Channel — 191
   - Self Pleasure — 193
   - Energy Attraction — 196
   - The Invitation Ceremony — 200
   - The Art of Orgasmic Creation — 204
   - Orgasmic Creation Ceremony — 210
   - Summary — 216
   - Applying the 4th Sacred Law to the Work Place — 217

9. Summing It All Up — 219

Resources and Offerings — 225

INTRODUCTION

MY WHY AND YOURS

MY BIG WHY behind this book, is a dream of sexual awareness and expression grounded in peacefulness and joy.

My vision is for teens and young adults to have access to sex education that teaches the beauty of sexuality, the sacredness of it, the power, the responsibility, the full sexual anatomy, conscious communication, and how to honor boundaries of self and others.

In my dream, everyone is safe, peaceful and living a joyful love life, spiritually, sexually and emotionally with or without a partner.

YOUR WHY FOR READING THIS BOOK...
When your Primal Sexual Body merges with your Divine Spirit Body from a space of peacefulness with

everyone from your past, it is a joy unlike any other.

* It is our Divine Design *

This book is a guide to take you there.

ABOUT THE TITLE

The word "Sacred" as defined in the Merriam Webster dictionary means "Devoted exclusively to one service or use" and "Highly valued and important." The Four Sacred Laws in this book are in devotion to who we are as Divine Beings inhabiting a physical Sexual Body.

A definition for the word "Law" is: "A rule or order that is advisable or obligatory to observe." Although not obligatory, it is advisable to observe and embody these Four Sacred Laws, and in doing so, you will experience greater well-being, expanded joy, deeper connection, and awakened ecstasy, with or without a partner.

SYMBOLISM

The cover of this book features the color orange, the color of our 2nd Chakra, the Sacral Chakra; the energy activation center for sexual and creative energy. Orange is associated with joy, warmth, creativity, health, happiness, balance, sexuality, freedom and expression.

Yellow is the color of the 3rd Chakra, the Solar Plexus. It is our power center and where we hold our emotions. Yellow is a color of happiness and enlightenment. The more we align with happiness, the more we are in our power.

The White Lotus Flower symbolizes enlightenment, beauty, purity, and power of knowledge.

WITH LOVE

This book is a culmination of wisdom from my life experience, relationships and from my own healing journey.

It's from my quest to understand the integral connection between my relationship with God/Spirit, and my sexual expression, and the beauty I found in that.

It is from receiving mentorship, research, and the experience of working with hundreds of private clients and facilitating thousands of workshop participants.

It's so beautiful to hold space for others as I witness them go through their transformation, moving from stress to calm, contraction to joy and open to a life of more pleasure.

I adore the breath, and I love to share how to activate it as an instrument to release unwanted emotion, to breathe more peace into the body and soul, to merge the sexual body with the spirit body, to expand physical pleasure and spiritual awakening.

I share this book with love. It is my prayer that this knowledge and wisdom will inspire healing and awakening as you implement it into your life. I'm not sharing anything new; I believe I am reminding you of what you already know on a soul level… your powerful truth as a Divine Spiritual Being living inside a Sexual Orgasmic Body.

Much love to you,
Jaitara

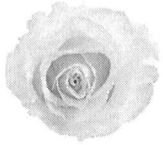

"When you feel a peaceful joy, that's when you are near truth." ~ Rumi

---

PART ONE

The JOURNEY *of* DISCOVERY

PRELUDE *to* THE FOUR SACRED LAWS

CHAPTER 1

The Day *of the* Grackle

The planting of the seed that eventually led to the birth of this book began in 1999. My full time career was acting and part time arts and crafts creations I sold at music festivals and gift shops. Back then, I never imagined that I would end up specializing in Sacred Sexuality, emotional healing and relationship coaching. I had never even heard of the term Sacred Sexuality or of Tantra.

I also have a gift in helping those at the end of their life leave their body with joy and peacefulness. At some point, I may even work as a Death Doula. Sexuality and death are more closely related than you may think. Each is a vehicle for being birthed into a new realm of existence. Each is orgasmic for the one who surrenders to love as they move through the experience.

The turning point for me was one day in 1999 when I recognized that the exploitation I experienced as a young teen was actually child abuse. This resulted in an emotional breakdown that quickly transformed into a breakthrough and an awakening that transcended my pain into wisdom. It was the beginning of my explorative journey of Sacred Sexuality and emotional healing.

Most people who knew me were unaware of the self-judgment I carried all those years leading to the day of my awakening. Until then, I never shared with anyone what had happened to me as a young teen, except for two men. One was my ex-husband and he responded in silence, which resulted in me staying silent, never speaking with him about it again. The other was a boyfriend who was raped when he was nine years old. Since his wounds never healed, with him it was a competition about whose wounds were deeper. This resulted in me never sharing this experience with anyone else until after that day in 1999, that I now call *The Day of the Grackle*.

I became skilled at giving off the appearance of having much more confidence than I actually did. My close friends knew something was off in my self-worth and emotional strength by the unhealthy choices I made in relationships. They just had no idea where it came from. After all, I was raised in a well-educated home with a loving mother in middle-class suburbia. The possibility of what I had actually been through was not on their radar.

THE AWAKENING

It is November 1999, I'm forty-two and living in Toronto, Canada. I'm standing on a subway platform and before me is a powerful sign from the Universe. It's an actual billboard on the wall of the other side of the subway

platform that says, "Teenage prostitution is child a
Suddenly I can't breathe. I am in shock. Staring at the sign, I am jolted awake to a truth I had not realized before this moment. You see, I was that child and before this moment, I just thought I was a "bad girl." Before this moment, I assumed everyone was better than me. Before this moment it hadn't occurred to me that what I experienced as a sixteen-year-old girl was sexual exploitation and abuse.

I don't remember the thirty-minute journey home from the subway station. Next thing I know, I am standing in my bathroom, looking out the window overlooking the backyard and the beautiful large evergreen tree. Suddenly twenty-seven years of repressed emotions are erupting out of me.

I am feeling the grief of losing my adolescence as memories of my past flash before me, with visions of the days when my body was sold for dollars, playing the role of a call girl when other girls my age were school girls and attending their prom.

I'm remembering the man who groomed my sixteen-year-old self for months, strategically activating my sexual energy while luring in my heart and luring me away from the safety of my home. Once he was sure I believed I was in love with him, he became my pimp. My anger is erupting as I remember how he tricked and manipulated me, controlling me through my love as he sold off my young body.

However, it is the rage that is most unbearable as for the first time in twenty-seven years I am waking up to the truth of what my junior high school principal had done. Suddenly I vividly remember that night in 1972 when I was sitting next to him on a bar stool in the Nova Scotian Hotel, at three years under legal drinking age.

I remember how he took me to a hotel with rooms that rent by the hour. I remember my petite body lying next to his large six-foot-plus body. I remember lying next to his wooden leg and the sensation of the hard wood touching my young naked body, as he told me he always thought I was sexy. (I attended his school between the ages of twelve to fourteen.) I remember him praising me on my new career choice as a child prostitute, saying, "This is a good choice for you. You'll be good at this."

I remember feeling the distortion of the moment, stuck in the reality of it, confused by his praise and guidance.

Now at this moment, looking out my bathroom window, I recognize the destructive impact of his words all those years ago. I recognize how I had seen my junior high school principal as an authority and father figure and this was his moment to rescue me, to protect me, to guide me. Instead, he made a choice I now recognize for the first time as child abuse.

These memories resurface and unfold in about twenty seconds, yet I feel stuck in time as my soul is being jolted awake. Each layer of memories overlapping one another, triggering the grief, the anger, and the rage, feeling like one debilitating collage of memories piercing the heart of my soul.

I'm gasping for breath as these emotions erupt out of me in a fraction of the time that it is taking for you to read these words. The impact is so intense, so painful that I feel like I am going to literally explode. I scream, "God please help me!"

The moment I call out these words, a bird flies from the east and lands on my back-patio railing. As if someone flicked a switch, I instantly become peaceful. I know this bird is a response from Spirit to my cry for help. I continue to stand and gaze out the window at this bird. I've never seen one like it before. It has the body of a dove, with black feathers that turn blue and purple iridescent from the sun's light. The bird stays just long enough for me to get a good look and then flies off to the west.

Spirit communicates with me through animals because they know I will go look it up. The moment the bird flies away, I run to get my *Animal Speak* book by Ted Andrews. I search the chapter on birds, looking for the bird on my patio and what message it has for me. I find it. The bird is a Grackle.

The teaching of the Grackle is to release emotional congestion from the past before it manifests into physical illness so you can move forward into the future. At this moment, the presence of Divine Spirit feels more tangible than ever before. I am in awe at the perfection of the timing of this message and give myself permission to continue to release the emotional congestion pouring out of me.

In Shamanism the East represents new life, birth, and creation. The West is affiliated with sunset. The direction of the setting sun represents a letting go of a limiting perspective. As we move into the darkness of night, it is a time to be like a Caterpillar and go within and cocoon where the past can be shed.

For two days, I stay home. I cry, I scream, I collapse on the floor. I sleep, I wake up and I do it again. I do not know about the breath work process I would eventually be certified to facilitate, otherwise, my purging would unfold within a couple of hours, but this is my experience and I embrace it. Through all of this, I never feel alone. I am acutely aware of Spirit watching over me, present with me, holding me in love.

After two days of intense emotional release, I feel a veil lift off of me. For the first time since the days when I was still a virgin, I feel myself falling in love with me again.

After these two days, I get on the phone and I call up all my friends and say, "Guess what happened to me as a teenager!" I finally felt liberated and free from the secret shame and self-judgment I had carried for so long, and my friends finally understood the source of my misaligned choices in men.

THE BLESSING OF IT ALL

By giving myself permission to express and purge my emotions, I opened to a new phase of emotional freedom in my life. After those two days, I became more sensitive to feeling layers of unworthiness in other women whom I previously would have seen as very confident. I also sensed that for most, this unworthiness was rooted in their sexual energy.

I still had more layers to heal within myself, but the emotional breakdown that happened on that Day of the Grackle quickly transformed into the breakthrough that planted the first seed of my desire to help other women heal their sexual wounds. It birthed my desire to support them in discovering a greater sense of self-worth and love. This work would later expand into working with men to do the same, and to supporting couples to deepen and expand their love and sexual intimacy.

Even through my years of hidden shame, sex was very pleasurable for me, with explosive orgasms. However, I felt a disconnect of my sexual body from my spiritual body. I compartmentalized them. I kept my spirituality in one box and my sexuality in another. I knew intuitively this is not how it is meant to be, so after that Day of the Grackle, I began a spiritual quest, exploring my connection between God and my sexuality.

The more I conversed with my Divine Team and merged my connection with God Source with my sexual expression, the more beautiful and expansive the physical pleasure became, and my connection to Source. This was years before I heard of Sacred Sexuality, yet my Sacred Sexual journey had begun.

This new relationship with Source was the beginning of my journey that eventually led to the discovery and unfolding of *The Four Sacred Laws of Sexual Enlightenment*.

THE HEALING CONTINUED

Years later, in 2004, I discovered the Holistic Rebirthing Breath facilitated by Mahara Brenna who later became my mentor. This breath healed and set free the remaining layers within me. I had tried other forms of breath work and although they were all powerful, this method was the most effective and was truly lasting. It cleared on a cellular level the emotional residue I had been carrying from my adolescence. It transmuted my pain to wisdom, lightness, aliveness, and wholeness.

In the early part of 2009, I was even contemplating taking my own life. I had just moved to a new home. In the house I lived in prior, I had some roommate situations gone horribly wrong that I believe were karmic experiences playing themselves out as I gave up my power... but that's another book, so I won't go into that story. I had been a Reiki Master Teacher for ten years by then and had been a practitioner of energy healing massage and sacred sexuality for four years. I believed I had cleared all the emotional residue from my adolescent abuse experience, but some final fragments were making their way to the surface.

I didn't identify the heaviness I was feeling at the time as residue from my adolescence. All I knew is that I wanted to go back home to the transcendental realm. One day I went into what I call emotional labor. I started wailing like a baby in the morning and two hours later it had not let up. So, I crawled across the floor on my hands and knees and reached for the Rebirthing audio Mahara had created and put it in my stereo and cranked up the volume and took myself through a Rebirthing session. One final surge of rage toward my junior high school principal purged out of me throughout the entire session as I breathed, screamed and beat the crap out of a pillow.

After this session, I fell asleep for two hours. When I woke up, it felt like I had lost a thousand pounds. I went from feeling heavy to lightness. The breath literally saved my life. That is why I am now a facilitator of this breath.

Shortly after that breath work session, I was taking a bath one day and I felt inspired to ask my Divine Team that any shadow and residue still stuck in my body all the way back to when I was in my mother's womb be removed from my body. Suddenly my body shook and thrashed about involuntarily just like a dog's body vigorously shakes after coming out of the water. I could see holes popping open in my body's energy field with beams of bright white light bursting through them.

It was like the energy clearing process of cord pulling. With cord pulling you envision where in your body you feel an energetic connection to a person or situation and you imagine the energetic connection is a cord. Then you wrap your hands around the cord and you pull it out by the root to clear yourself of the energy. This thrashing about in the bathtub was like that, only it was happening by itself at warp speed all over me. It was like dark energetic cords were popping out of my body with white divine light filling the space beaming out of me where the cord once was. It lasted for about ten seconds. It was one of the most powerful, beautiful, unusual, and very cool energy clearing experiences I've ever experienced.

We are Divine Eternal Beings. At the core, we are pure love. Our bodies are miracles of creation. The way our Sexual Body works in harmony with our Spiritual Body is how Creation intended or it would not be possible. It is our Divine Design.

If thinking of yourself as a Divine being does not resonate with your belief system, then maybe this book is not for you. If this does resonate with you, by remembering and embracing your Divinity, you free yourself from feelings of less than. Because you exist, that makes you worthy of all the goodness, pleasure, love and abundance this life has to offer.

You are an extension of God Source Energy expressing as you. You are Creator and more powerful than you may know. Your body is a temple. You are an exquisite gift. As you free yourself from the emotional wounds of your past, the more liberated you become to express the true essence of you, and the more the rest of us get to experience and celebrate the gift of you.

When your primal sexual body merges with your Divine spirit body from a space of peacefulness with everyone and everything from your past, it is a joy unlike any other. It is your Divine Design. It is the intention of creation.

THE DAY OF THE GRACKLE 13

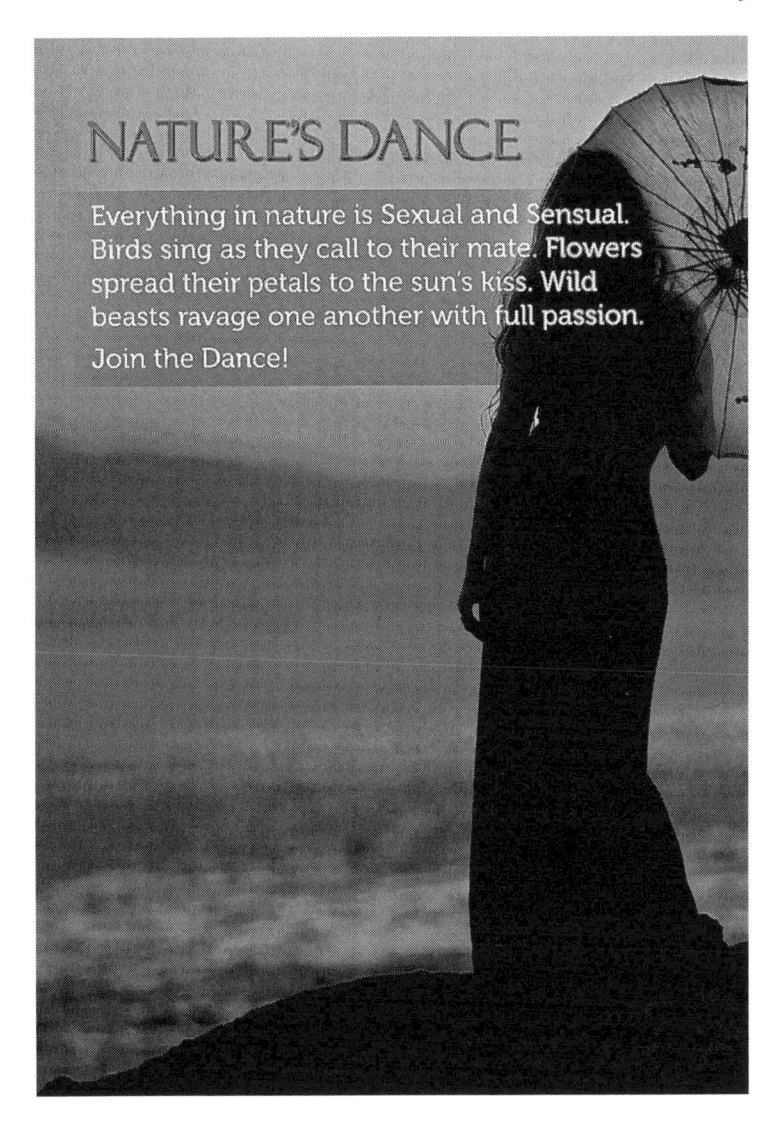

NATURE'S DANCE

Everything in nature is Sexual and Sensual. Birds sing as they call to their mate. Flowers spread their petals to the sun's kiss. Wild beasts ravage one another with full passion.

Join the Dance!

CHAPTER 2

Bear Medicine

THE VISION

The first time I introduced these Four Sacred Laws was in 2012 through a Video Series. Since then the creation of this book remained a strong vision in my soul. In October 2014, I planned a trip into the country to write my first words.

I envisioned myself starting the book in a cabin surrounded by nature. In this vision, I saw a wood stove in the cabin. Little did I know how beautifully the Universe would orchestrate this vision into reality. The following is the story of how I began the writing of this book and the magical significance that black bears would play in the unfolding of my journey.

I searched a few home rental websites, with determination to find a cottage with a wood stove and trees surrounding it. I love the aroma of a wood fireplace and the sound of a crackling fire. It inspires me. It felt important for me to find a fireplace that was a freestanding wood stove, versus a fireplace built into the wall. I would soon understand this was my Divine Team guiding me to the perfect cabin to begin my book.

After researching all of my options, I found a quaint cabin with a wood burning stove as the heat source in a small town called Spences Bridge, three hours inland from Vancouver. The photos on the website revealed this little cottage with a red door and a cozy living room where the stove stood. It had a raised mattress and throw cushions against the living room window that can be a window seat or spare bed. There was a lovely bedroom with a large picture window overlooking the backyard.

I booked the cabin for ten days to give a good kick-start to the book. I envisioned myself sitting propped up against the pillows at the window seat writing. There were large evergreen trees outside both the front and backyard windows. Across the street from the front yard was the Thompson River with train tracks running alongside it. The backyard was private with a tall wooden fence.

The cabin was magical. One of my favorite features was the outdoor claw foot bathtub with a garden hose that ran only hot water into the tub. In this tub, I could enjoy outdoor hot baths overlooking the yard and the mountains that were the backdrop of this town. The population of the town is approximately 250 people. Many residents are descendants of the Thompson River People, the indigenous First Nations People of the Interior Salish language group.

I was also intrigued by the fact that Jean, the owner of the cottage, shared with me there was a possibility of an occasional sighting of a black bear walking by the cabin. Being an animal lover, I was hoping to catch a glimpse of one while there.

Jean told me that her cabin was built by well-known author, John Alexander Teit. He is famous for doing intensive field research and for writing major publications on the Thompson Natives. John Teit was a contributor to a five-year project called the Jesup North Pacific Expedition. Teit authored four of the twenty-seven JNPE publications that ended up in the American Museum of *Natural History's Memoirs* in New York. In the late 1800s, author John Teit built the very cabin I would start my book in, to write his books.

My vision and desire for a wood stove was Divine intervention guiding me to this magical author's cabin for the experience I would have with the bears. It was the only cabin I could find within reasonable driving distance in the countryside of British Columbia with the deal breaker wood stove.

THE JOURNEY THERE

It's the morning of the day I am leaving for the cabin. I'm packed and ready for my ten day recluse in Spences Bridge. I pick up the phone and call my host to let her know I'm starting my three hour drive there. She says, "You must have powerful energy. There is a mother bear with her two cubs up the tree right in front of the house. I've never seen them there before. When you arrive, look up the tree before getting out of your car. If you see the bears in the tree, then come around to the back entrance. You don't want to disturb a mama bear with cubs."

I am hoping they will still be there when I arrive, so I can get a close view from inside the cabin of this precious family.

During the first couple hours of driving, I am surrounded by views of lush trees British Columbia is known for. I didn't realize until this trip that Spences Bridge is at the edge of the only area in Canada called a desert, known as the Okanagan Desert. It's not really a desert, rather a shrub-steppe area. It's still unique countryside compared to the rest of the province. As I get closer, the trees on the mountains thin out, changing the landscape into that of a much drier climate.

As I'm driving through this new landscape getting closer to my destination, a strange feeling is coming over me. I am suddenly very emotional with tears streaming down my face. I feel the pain of the women before me who lived on this land. I feel the ancestors, the grandmothers speaking to me, telling me how important my book is, that for too many generations women were suppressed and shamed for their sexuality. I feel how for years they yearned to be expressed and honored. I feel the ancestors supporting me on this journey.

I suddenly burst into the *Strong Women's Song*, an Ojibwe drumming song I learned while immersed in the Ojibwe community in Ontario. I'm now singing loudly from the depths of my soul while driving with my hands drumming on the steering wheel as the tears keep streaming down my face. What a profound, powerful and a tangible experience this is, feeling the ancestors in the Spirit realm connecting and communicating with me.

THE BEAR CABIN

When I arrive at the cabin, there is no mama bear in the tree. Before I have a chance to feel disappointed that I missed out on seeing them, Jean tells me there is a rather large male black bear sleeping just outside the window. I couldn't resist, so I look out through the window facing the side of the house. Laying there sleeping is an extremely large black bear.

A fence separates the cabin from the neighbor's property no more than six feet away, with a water heater next to the rear of the cabin blocking a path to the backyard, leaving the front yard as the only way in and out of this side patch. This makes a perfect little cubby cave space for the bear to snooze in.

The windowpane is open, as I approach it the bear wakes up and hears me through the screen. Gently I say. "Hello bear!"

He lifts his head and looks at me. He is only about five feet from the window. "You are so beautiful!" I say.

I continue to converse in this way as he stays laying on his side with his head up looking at me with what appeared to be equal intrigue. Then he snorts. Now, I hadn't done my research on black bear behavior yet, but I intuitively know this snort is his way of warning me to back off so he can go back to sleep. I quickly oblige, slowly lowering the windowpane, with my heart pounding a little quicker now while feeling a deep gratitude for the presence of my majestic neighbor. Little do I know, this is just an intro to my Bear Medicine experience in Spences Bridge.

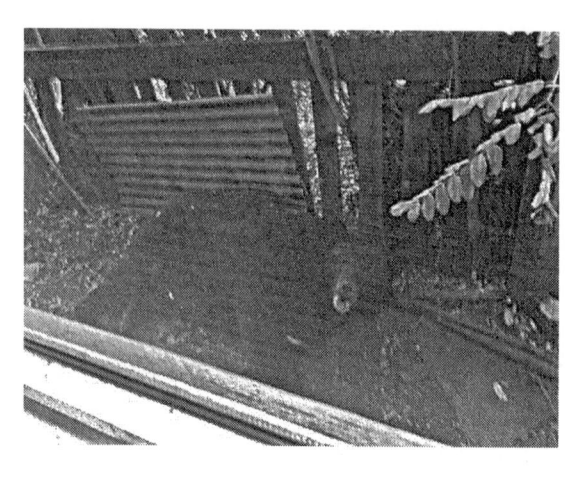

My new Bear friend

There are several apple and pear trees on many properties in this town. Many homes are summer homes, not occupied during the fall and winter months, so there is an abundance of fresh fruit for the picking by local bears, both on the trees and on the ground below them, making it a feast in the fall months just before hibernation time.

The proper way to behave when you come face to face with a black bear is to stand your ground, hold eye contact and back up slowly. However, sometimes, running is more appropriate. This is something I receive a powerful lesson in, as you'll discover soon.

The Big Man Bear continues to be my cabin mate camping out beside the cabin. He sleeps during the day then leaves at dusk to go wandering for food and feast on the local fruit. I love his presence. I love gazing out the window at his beautiful self, sometimes sleeping on his back with his big bear paws up in the air. I feel so blessed.

Each morning I love bathing in the hot tub of water in the backyard, gazing at the beautiful view of the tall evergreen tree against the yard fence and the mountains beyond. It's now day three at the cabin and while in the tub I discover that I am not alone. Someone is witnessing my bath ritual. It is the Man Bear, out from his sleeping spot and up in the evergreen tree.

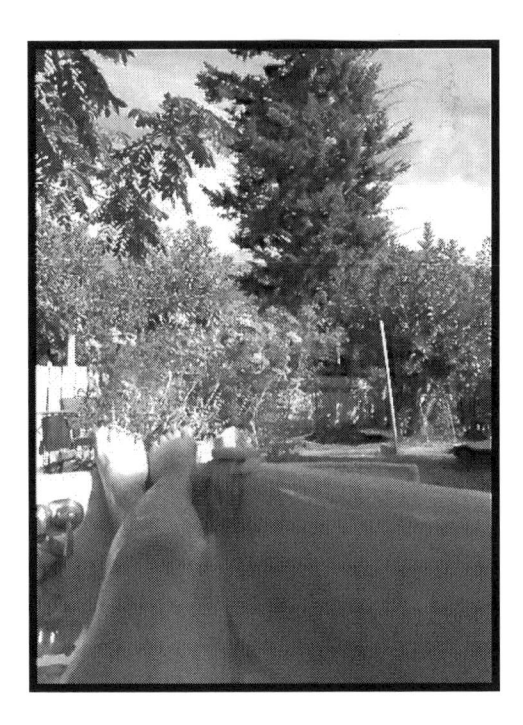

Morning bath with view of the bear tree

I suddenly feel compelled to sing one of my favorite Sanskrit chants, *Hey Ma Durga* by Donna DeLory. This chant is an invocation of the Divine Mother. I'm singing away and Bear is sitting as still as can be in the tree. With singing not being one of my gifts, I'm not sure if my singing is scaring him or soothing him. As soon as I stop singing, he climbs up higher. I feel so at ease and safe sharing my space with the Big Man Bear.

It's later in the day now and I am walking down the town street and I see a small cluster of people just a few doors down from my cabin standing in the road looking up at the trees. There, high in a tree in a neighbor's yard, is the Mama Bear and her two cubs, looking at us looking at her and her babies. What a beautiful sight. She is calm as she sees we maintain a respectful distance. The yard's fence separates us, as well as the height of the tree, contributing to her sense of safety.

So here I am hanging out, taking photos and videos of this beautiful family. Then, one of the local Natives, a Nlaka'pamux man walks up and joins us. Laughing he says, "I came to watch the tourists watch the bears." I'm sure he is also making sure we maintain a good level of respect for our wild friends.

Once done with the bear viewing, I took myself out for dinner at the only diner in town and now I'm walking back home to my cabin. I suddenly stop in my tracks as I see my Big Man Bear in the next-door neighbor's yard as I'm passing by. There is no fence around this yard to separate us. He is chowing down on some apples. He stops and looks me in the eyes. I maintain my gaze into his. He turns and runs off in the other direction. Whew! That was cool!

Now it's day four. It's morning and I'm out in the backyard with my little dog Quincy. She's having her morning backyard walk about before I get ready for my bath. There up in the tree is my Man Bear again... or so I think. Feeling familiar with him now, I call out, "Hello bear! Nice to see you again. Stay up in the tree, I'm taking my doggie for a pee!"

Suddenly I hear loud growls and the tree branches rapidly breaking. Bear is bolting down the tree. Instantly I realize, this is not my Man Bear. This is the Mama Bear, and she is in fierce mode. My Quincy, oblivious to the danger, lets out a scream from the shock of me grabbing her up by the scruff of her neck. I bolt into the house through the back-yard door. This is one of those times, you don't stop to make eye contact with a black bear. You run!

I am now safely in the house and I run into the bedroom to look out the picture window that overlooks the yard. There I see mama bear jump off the tree and onto the other side of the fence. Her cubs must be there waiting for her. This is one day I will not be taking a bath in the yard.

It's later now and dusk is setting in. I go into the bedroom and look out the picture window and there is mama with her two babies wandering around in the backyard. She comes so close to the house walking right under the window where I am standing. If it were open I could reach my hand out and touch her.

The cubs are playfully exploring the backyard and the back patio. Mama joins them on the patio and stands up on her hind legs to check out an animal skull that is décor over the back door, showing me the grandeur of her size and grace. I try to take photos but the light is too dark, and I know a flash will alarm her. I also know that the picture window will not stop her from bursting into the house to protect her cubs from the threat she believes I am if she knows I am here. So, I stand still in the dark in awe watching the family romp around until they wander off.

The locals told me there is also a lone cub in town whose mother was killed by a train a few days ago. In front of the cabin is a tree swing with a big stuffed toy bear sitting on it. It's now day five, the day after my experience with the mama and her cubs. As I sit in the front window seat, I see the lone cub playfully run up to the swing. What a precious one he is as he paws at the stuffed bear on the swing until it falls on the ground. He gives it a sniff and realizing it's not a real baby bear and goes bouncing down the street.

I heard the locals say he likely would not live through the winter without a mother to guide him and take care of him. I hope that a wildlife protection service will come to rescue him, but apparently, the community leaves nature to take its course and won't interfere with the natural unfolding of the wild.

It's now day six and my Big Man Bear is gone. All that is left are large mounds of bear poop. Maybe he moved on to find a cleaner area to sleep in. I feel the lack of his presence and I miss him.

I feel so honored by this time in the cabin, the presence of Bear and the medicine teachings they bring. I got two chapters started while in the bear cabin, Sacred Law One and Two. I did not write as many hours as I thought I would. I realize much of this journey was for me to go within into deep reflection.

I was also there to receive the profound message and energy of the grandmother ancestors. I was there to experience a deep connection to Bear and the teachings they brought me. I was there for my own soul healing and soul-searching that was necessary at this time to step into the power of this book.

BEAR MEDICINE & SEXUAL ENLIGHTENMENT

So, what is the relevance of my experience with the bears in relation to this book? What does bear medicine have to do with *The Four Sacred Laws of Sexual Enlightenment*? How does it connect with my emotional experience in the car when I heard the messages of the ancestors?

In Ted Andrew's *Animal Speak* book he writes about how the hibernation period of Bear teaches us to go within, to meditate and explore your inner sanctum to find your answers. He shares that Bear teaches us to tap into our inner wisdom and bring it out into the world.

My journey that led to writing this book was deep and meditative. I spent many hours in prayer and communicating with Spirit in my quest to understand how my relationship with God merges with my sexual expression, and how to help others do the same. The messages I received from the ancestors on the day on my drive to Spences Bridge was a powerful confirmation of the importance of me bringing this wisdom into the world to share with others.

The Mama Bear is known for her fierce protection of her cubs. She also teaches courage and confidence to her cubs. The Mama Bear teaches her cubs to survive and thrive in the wild, while also teaching them to have very strong boundaries.

I do not have children, but I see the welfare of our youth as a responsibility that belongs to all of us. Whether you are a parent or not, the children are our responsibility and we must be fierce in our protection of them. The greatest wounding that children experience is abuse. Sexual abuse among girls is the highest form of abuse endured. Boys experience this trauma as well. We are failing the youth at this time by the human trafficking and sex slavery that still exists in this world, and by the lack of conscious sex education. We live in a time when both boys and girls are turning to porn to learn about sex.

The ancestors spoke to me about protecting the daughters and sons from the same pain and wounding that those before them endured. By providing more complete guidance for children about sexuality, we can protect them from unnecessary wounding. This does not mean we shelter them. The youth need conscious sex education that teaches the full anatomy as well as the beauty of sex, the sacredness, the power, the responsibility, mindful communication and how to honor their boundaries. Imagine this as their legacy.

In this book, I share my wisdom and knowledge as a guide for you to heal and merge your connection to the Divine with your sexual expression. As adults, we must take responsibility for healing our wounds and for gaining sexual alignment for our own well-being, and also so we can teach by example and create a new legacy for our youth.

If you have a healthy relationship with your sexuality and you are fulfilled with the pleasure of it, then perfect. Maybe the reason you are reading this book is to take your pleasure to new heights, to reach a higher level of awakened ecstasy and to gain new inspiration and knowledge.

Bear is also strongly connected to trees. Here is a quote from the *Animal Speak* book: *"The tree is a powerful and ancient symbol, just like the bear. It is a natural antenna, linking the Heavens and the Earth. Different trees do have different meanings, but in general, it represents knowledge. It is a symbol of fertility, of things that grow."*

Sexual Enlightenment is also about linking the Heavens and the Earth. It is the merging of who we are as Divine Eternal Beings and our connection to God Source, with who we are as Earthly Physical Beings. It is the merging of our Spiritual body with our Sexual body. We are conduits between the two realms, like an antenna. When we do this consciously, we experience a whole new realm of Spiritual and Sexual ecstasy. Sexual energy is also how we fertilize the seed within the womb that creates life. How beautiful when this fertilization takes place while integrated with spiritual connection and love.

Here is another quote from the *Animal Speak* book:

"All bears have a great fondness for honey. Honey is the natural sweetness of life. It is usually found in the hives, located in trees, again reflecting a connection between bears and trees. It is a reminder for those with this totem to go within to awaken the power, but only by bringing it out into the open and applying it will the honey of life be tasted."

As Bear's love of honey reminds us to savor the sweetness of life, savor the beauty, pleasure, and sweetness of that which gives you life… your sexuality.

When we embrace this sweetness, we are most powerful. It is time as a society for us to shatter the illusion and distortion of sexual exploitation, shame, judgment, and contraction and instead embody and reclaim the truth of our Divine Design... our primal fire merged with our Divine light, and the sweetness of that. It is your birthright. It is what Creation intended. It's the legacy we owe to the next generation.

I am so grateful for the Bear Medicine teachings and their contribution to my journey of sexual enlightenment.

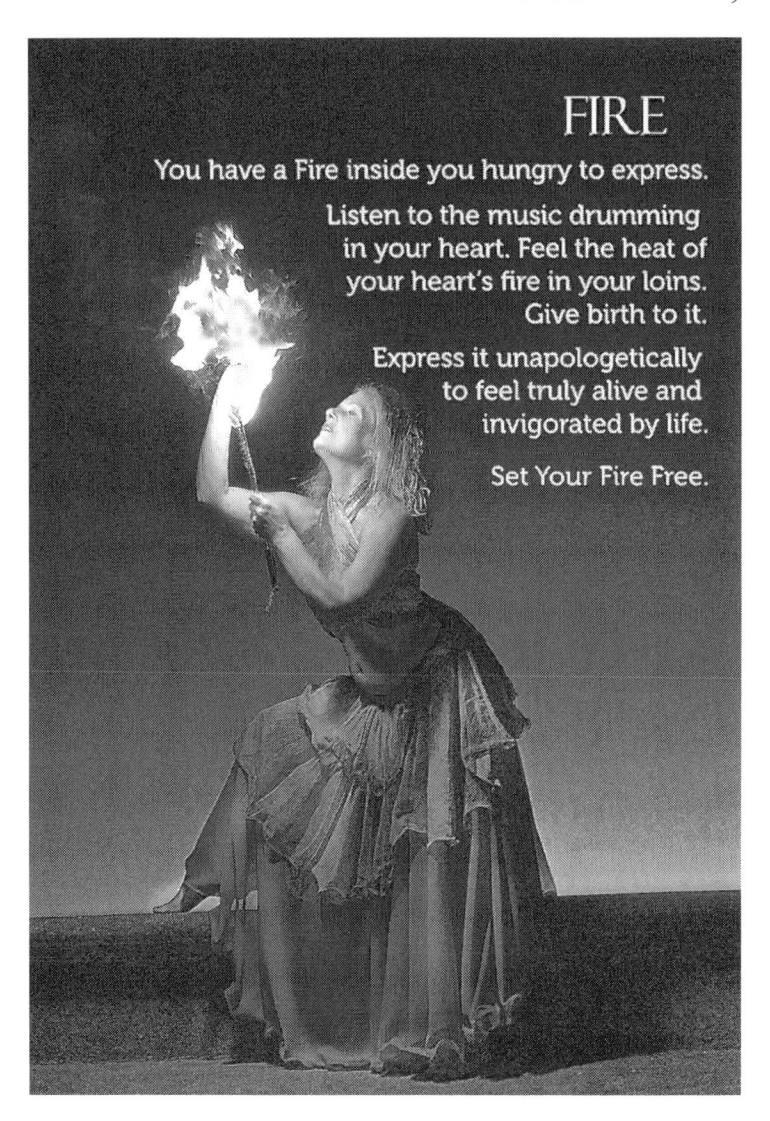

BEAR MEDICINE 29

FIRE

You have a Fire inside you hungry to express.

Listen to the music drumming in your heart. Feel the heat of your heart's fire in your loins. Give birth to it.

Express it unapologetically to feel truly alive and invigorated by life.

Set Your Fire Free.

CHAPTER 3

History *and* Herstory

"Put away your pointless taboos and restrictions on Sexual Energy, rather help others to truly understand its wonder and to channel it properly."
~ *God, channeled by Neale Donald Walsch*

HISTORY & HERSTORY OF SEXUAL SHAME

Approximately one out of every three women have experienced sexual assault or harassment. Men not as much, but it is a reality for them as well. What about you? Have you had a sexual assault or harassment experience? Besides past lifetime experiences, we are also affected by the collective experiences of society. As we look at how the societal perspective around sexuality has unfolded through time, we can observe the big picture and the truth within that.

The following information has been passed down through generations and appeared as a vision to many. I believe on a soul level it is true and beautiful. Tune into your soul's wisdom and decide for yourself.

There was a time in history when the spiritual gathering places were Priestess temples. I like to call this *herstory*. These Priestesses were healers and confidants, deeply honored for the role they played in the community. They understood the integral connection of sexual and spiritual energy, honoring sexual energy as a sacred gift from God. Some Priestesses specialized in sexual energy as a form of healing and medicine. When the men returned from battle, they would enter such temples and these Priestesses would bathe them and use sexuality as a healing modality to remove the energy frequency of war out of the warriors, so they could go back home to their families, and not carry the energy of battle home with them.

Priestess temples were eventually destroyed and churches were built on the land where they once stood. Women were then forbidden to practice all types of medicine. Years later, the witch burnings began. Women felt forced to point fingers and blame one another out of fear for their own lives. Women who displayed signs of enjoyment of sexual expression were accused of consorting with the devil.

SEXUAL PRIESTESS

"A Priestess knows that everything is Sacred.
She holds the wisdom of Heaven and Earth, honors women as Sisters,
walks the path of compassion, self-care and embodied beauty. A Sexual
Priestess awakens healing through Sacred Sexual Expression.
Embrace your inner Sexual Priestess."
~ Sacred Sexual Enlightenment Wisdom Cards

Single women with land were in great danger during the inquisition. One man was employed to seek them out, others to arrest them, and others to possess their land. The land and property were sold and everyone shared in the profits. Witch burning was a big business and it went on for three to four hundred years, yet it is barely mentioned in our history books.

For a couple thousand years, the patriarchal religions have worked to split our sexuality from our spirituality. We became sexually repressed. It's quite a master plan when you think about it. How better to control a society than to inflict guilt and shame around the very energy that creates us and the energy we cannot resist, while suppressing women who are the bearers of life.

The only female sexual role models that women had to identify with were the virgin and the whore, with nothing between. Throughout time, a whore has been seen as a woman who is less than and shunned by society, instead of being recognized as a woman who has made her own choices or was forced to make choices she didn't want to. Some hurt themselves by working in a profession that doesn't make them happy. They deserve our compassion, not judgment. Those who work in the sex trade today and enjoy their work also deserve our compassion, acceptance, and recognition that they too are worthy of all that is good.

We were a good girl or a bad girl. This is a wound passed on from mother to daughter for generations. This has affected men equally. When there is a wounding of the Feminine in society it is also a reflection of the wounded Feminine that lives within men.

The Priestess archetype is in all religions throughout

time, yet it has been lost in our psyches for a few thousand years. It's only recently this archetype became more popular to where it is even trendy. Priestess groups and circles are surfacing all over the planet with women feeling called on a soul level to discover this aspect of themselves.

The following piece of writing was given to me by my friend and numerologist, Jan Nieuwenhuis. He is an avid historian. He shares this information from memory of his own extensive research. As you read this, feel how the words resonate with you. As you read this, feel how Jan's words resonate with you... or not. I suspect some readers may even be offended, while others will resonate deeply.

"In the days of Mother Mary and Mary Magdalene, "Mary" was not a name. It was a title denoting a 'virgin priestess attached to the temple.' Royalty is passed along through the genes of the female, not the male. The role of virgin priestess to the temple is a very important one. Throughout history it has generally been men who have performed the day-to-day, mundane, regular functions of the king, taxation, war, governing, but it is the queen who gave them the legitimacy to do so. Of interest, consider how the queen is in fact the most powerful piece on the chessboard, not the king.

Mary the mother, was impregnated by a priest of the temple representing the holy line of Levi. The offspring Jesus, not of immaculate conception as claimed by the church but born in the regular normal everyday manner, was given to Mary to be raised until the age of 7 with the help of a surrogate father, a step-father if you will. That person was Joseph. He was just a convenient guardian. That was his only role.

At the age of 7 Jesus was returned to the temple to be instructed by his biological father, the priest. When in the bible it is stated that, 'Jesus went to the temple to see his father,' it is to see his actual flesh and blood father, not the white bearded figure in the sky that many people call God. This is where the myth of the 'Son of God' was born. He was no such thing. In fact the 'Son of God' title is an obfuscation of the older deification of Apollo, he being the 'Sun of God,' a remnant of a much older sun worship cult.

That myth of the 'Son of God' was cemented into place in the years 100 to 300 because it effectively shut out any offspring Jesus could have had with Mary Magdalena. And, there was indeed offspring, two boys by the information that has been passed down.

The marriage recounted in the bible during which Jesus reportedly turned the water into wine, was in fact his own wedding. Mary Magdalena, another priestess of the temple was his wife. That duplication of names shows a continuity of what may be termed 'Grail Priestesses'; Mary the mother, Mary the wife, both performing the function of mother to royal offspring.

Jesus was in fact a legitimate king living in hiding during times of Roman occupation.

After the crucifixion, Mary and the two boys left Palestine and ended up in Marseilles, in Gaul, where a fragment of followers thereafter created a small municipality. Much later in time after the fall of the oppressive Roman Empire, that area formed the core of rise of the Merovingian kings of early Gaul. Kings who had a mystical, mysterious and a seemingly mythological origin.

They were usurped in 751 by Pepin, the 'Mayor of the Palace' to the last governing Merovingian king. He was given the backing of the pope who had a personal vested interest to suppress if not to actually exterminate the lineage of the flesh and blood Christ in favor of their contrived Christ, who was too 'holy' to ever have children. The church then coroneted Pepin's son, Charlemagne, later he was elevated to the status Emperor by the same papacy in the year 800.

Neither Pepin nor Charlemagne had an ounce of the so-called Holy

Blood. Queen Elizabeth is descended from Charlemagne. That's why Charles is such a common royal name.

The true bloodline has been reduced to the status of breeding stock. Diana was of that stock. The unicorn, a symbol of the fertility of Christ, is literally chained to the ground in the British Coat of Arms. The chains may be readily seen by anyone who takes the trouble to look.

The true king lives in obscurity in Scotland where James was an important name in their line of kings. James was the brother of Jesus and Jesus's next of kin regarding the passing on of the kingship while the children of Jesus grew to maturity under the care of their mother, the Magdalena, the Grail Queen."

If you would like to dive into researching the writings of this history/herstory in more depth, the information can be found in *The Hirem Key*, by Robert Lomas and Christopher Knight, published in 1996. Other books that Jan recommends that dive into the lineage of Jesus Christ, Mother Mary and Mary Magdalene are *The Holy Blood, Holy Grail* by Baigent, Lincoln and Leigh. Published in 1982. There is also *Bloodline of the Holy Grail, the Hidden Lineage of Jesus Revealed*, Published in 1989 and *Genesis of the Grail Kings* (1999) by Laurence Gardner.

I am an initiated and ordained High Priestess. What does this mean in modern day times and how does one become initiated? Priestess consciousness teaches us to live our lives in a sacred way in service to the world. She recognizes all women as Sisters and does not partake in gossip or competition against other women. A Priestess is a woman who offers her gifts in service. She is a woman who holds the wisdom of the connection between the Spiritual realm and the Earth, who longs to express herself in the temple of her life. She is a woman trained in performing sacred ceremony. A Priestess is dedicated to life affirming values. She empowers, teaches and guides change on all levels. A Priestess walks the feminine path of self-care, beauty and sacred sexuality.

I went through a two-part year and a half extensive journey with my circle of Priestess sisters, facilitated by Anyaa McAndrew, a High Priestess and Bishop of the Madonna Ministry. We explored the deepest part of ourselves. We explored our shadow side, our inner darkness and looked directly into this aspect of ourselves and embraced it with love. By holding this aspect of ourselves in the light of love, we render it powerless.

During part-two, our High Priestess journey, we explored the conscious connection between our spiritual paths, our political beliefs, our sexuality, and our money stories. This connection is also recognized as the path of the Magdalene Priestess, uniting sexuality, heart, and vision. As we emerged as Priestesses at the end of the first part of our journey together, we had the option to be ordained into the Madonna Ministry. I chose that option.

Magdalene is recognized as the Beloved of Christ by all modern day Priestess lineages and circles. She is also recognized as a teacher and advocate for the Divine Feminine. She lived during a time when women were stoned to death for speaking in public. We've come a long way since then and women are finally finding their voice and the courage to speak their truth unapologetically. The Me Too Movement is an eruption of this.

At times women can take on characteristics that could be described as downright vicious, back biting and undermining. At the root of this behavior is always an unresolved wound that is showing at the surface as a projection. This is very prevalent in some of the reality TV shows that sensationalize conflict between women, dramatizing it and promoting it to increase their ratings, ultimately feeding a lower form of consciousness. It is disempowering for the women who engage in this activity, and can lead to the men who love them having distorted perceptions.

Women projecting judgments onto one another is toxic, and can create a split between the inner feminine and masculine, especially when the judgment is supported by the masculine. When this happens, it can feel unsafe and cause a block in the heart energy, ultimately affecting the ability or inability to experience a healthy relationship.

When I work with women, early on I guide them to connect with their inner healthy Divine masculine, who witnesses without judgment and provides safety. Once the self-judgment ceases, they step into greater self-worth and self-love. This evolves into feeling safe to express more of their feminine essence for themselves and toward one another. As women connect with the healthy masculine essence within themselves, they attract men as friends and lovers who are the embodiment of the healthy masculine.

When men connect with inner feminine qualities of compassion and nurturing, whether consciously or not, they attract the same in women they connect with; and can experience healthier trusting relationships with other men.

Instead of judging, blaming, or trying to reason through argument, if instead we apply understanding through empathy, a situation can change and evolve with love.

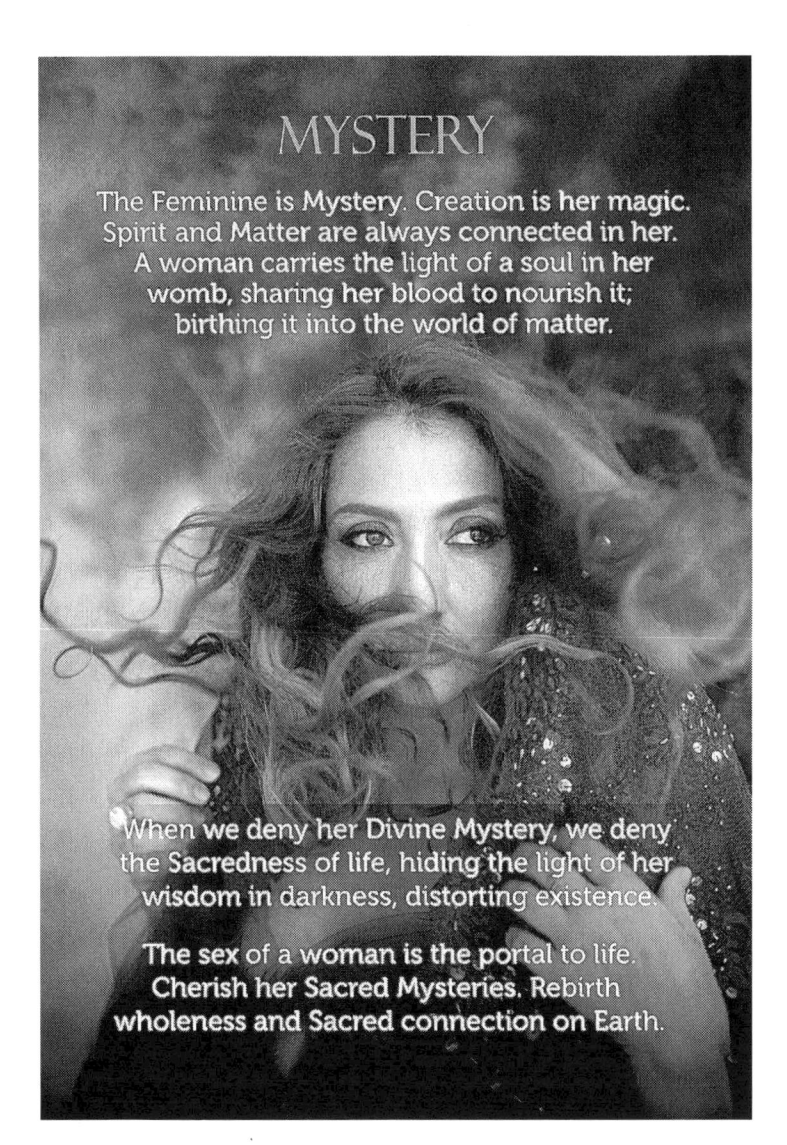

HISTORY AND HERSTORY 39

MYSTERY

The Feminine is Mystery. Creation is her magic.
Spirit and Matter are always connected in her.
A woman carries the light of a soul in her
womb, sharing her blood to nourish it;
birthing it into the world of matter.

When we deny her Divine Mystery, we deny
the Sacredness of life, hiding the light of her
wisdom in darkness, distorting existence.

The sex of a woman is the portal to life.
Cherish her Sacred Mysteries. Rebirth
wholeness and Sacred connection on Earth.

Shame and guilt around our sexuality have disempowered all of us. Both women and men have been affected by this damaging history and herstory throughout time. By recognizing this and going to the source, we can cast a light on this shadow aspect and transform how we feel about ourselves and how we see one another. It's time to remember and own the fact that our sexuality is integrally connected to our spiritual self. It is our creative force. Honor it as the Sacred Gift it is. Embrace your wholeness as a Divine being living in a primal sexual orgasmic body temple. This is your truth, Beloved.

When you entered puberty, were you taught the sacredness of sexual energy? Were you taught to honor your own Divinity and the Divinity in those you felt attracted to? How blessed you were if this was your reality. Or, did you feel you fit into one of two sexual categories, that you were either good or bad? Were you made to feel shameful of your sexuality or scolded if you were caught touching your own genitals? So much wounding has taken place simply through poor sexual guidance.

At the core of all wounds is a girl or boy not knowing they are good enough. They don't recognize the truth of who they are. We are born wanting to give love and be loved. When boys and men disrespect girls and women, they are also disrespecting the feminine energy within themselves. When girls and women disrespect and judge men, they are also judging the masculine within themselves. The more aware we are of our own Divinity, the more we see it in one another, we open ourselves to greater compassion, love, peacefulness, wisdom, and connection.

AFRICAN HERSTORY

An African woman named Efua Dorkenoo, author of *Cutting the Rose* brings great awareness to the subject of female genital mutilation. She shares stories of the days from her great-grandmother in Zambia when the girls were taken into huts for two weeks upon entering puberty. The women elders taught them everything about their sexuality and how to honor their body. They were given wooden models to practice on. The elders would lie on top of the girls and pretend to be the man, teaching them how to move their hips and adopt the best positions for the most pleasure. At the end of the two weeks, when these girls returned into the community, they felt special and clearly understood their sexual energy and how to honor it.

Dorkenoo shares that girls given this kind of education at puberty exude a confidence in themselves and a deep respect for their own sexuality. She says, *"It gives them a sense of power in which they are taught not to abuse. These girls don't tend to be promiscuous. Sexuality is their gift from God. They may flaunt it in the way they walk, but they will save the best of what the elders have taught them for their man."*

I don't expect the grandmothers of today would do the same, although I personally would love it if they would. Imagine what a difference it would make if all young people were educated about sexuality in such an open, complete and truthful manner.

In the movie *Avatar*, the native women were practically nude, yet nothing was exploitive in how they were portrayed. The men and women lived together in harmony, honoring one another, connecting all that is physical to the Divine. Those who saw this movie were touched by this because we know in our hearts this is our highest way of being and co-existing.

MUTILATION OF THE MASCULINE

When we hear about genital mutilation of the feminine, most of us cringe in disgust at the Barbarianism. The fact is, genital mutilation of the masculine has been around for thousands of years and still exists in North America and other continents. It is more commonly called circumcision. It's been happening for so long that it's become an accepted medical practice that many parents agree to just because it is something that is done. I believe it is time for this history to change.

Circumcision reduces male sexual pleasure. It became common practice during a time when regular bathing was considered impractical, so they cut the foreskin to contribute to hygiene. It was also done as a method to discourage masturbation. If you research you will find many other reasons circumcision became a common practice in various cultures and civilizations. None of these reasons make sense in today's modern world.

Circumcision is genital mutilation. It's done to an infant child whose first experience of being touched on their genitals is one of extreme pain and confinement. He is bound to a table unable to move as they cut him. How does inflicting this trauma serve the boy child? It is time to leave this barbaric practice in our history. It's time to stop cutting the penises of infant children and allow their bodies to grow and develop as creation intended.

MY PERSONAL HERSTORY

I am a certified *Cuddle Party*® facilitator. One reason I was drawn to this is because it teaches proper communication and honoring boundaries regarding touch, as well learning how to say "no" and be comfortable using "no" as a complete sentence. When saying "no" feels difficult, it's because we feel a need to explain our "no," justify our "no", or we worry about hurting the other person's feelings with our "no".

Saying "no" was something I felt incapable of doing in my younger years. I've discovered this is the case for many young girls and women. Boys and men also struggle with this, but from my personal experience, it is much more prevalent in the feminine. Sometimes, as a teen and young woman I said "yes," but I was screaming "NO" on the inside. The word would not come out.

My father was a goodhearted man but a weak father figure. Expressing feelings was very difficult for him. Only twice in my life I heard him speak the words "I love you" and he did not know how to teach me boundaries. Because of my difficulty saying "no" and my longing for a father to express love for me, to tell me what to do and to guide me, I looked outside of the home for what I wanted from my father. What I experienced was the distorted masculine, pretending to care, good at telling me what to do, but not for my higher good. This led to the sexual exploitation I experienced that I shared in the previous chapter, *The Day of the Grackle*.

Like most abuse victims, I blamed myself. It's one thing to be a victim, but as time passes, there is a turning point where we go from being a victim to playing the victim. Recognizing this is the first step to healing and liberating yourself from wounds of the past.

My story is mild compared to many and all it takes to shift the statistics of sexual abuse and harassment is for the youth to have strong role models, guidance and accurate knowledge from the adult men and women in their lives at home, and in their community.

ME TOO/TIME'S UP

During the writing of this book, the Me Too Movement surfaced, as well as the corruption in Hollywood that led to all women in the film business coming together for change, initiating the phrase, "Time's Up." We live in a powerful time in history and herstory with an opportunity to rise above the distortion and misalignment that results from the residue of our past.

The majority of women and some men reading this book have a Me Too story. Well, I agree. Time's up! We are better than that. When women are honored, everyone flourishes. When women come together as sisters versus succumbing to manipulation and competition, we are empowered beyond measure. When men stand up embodying the king that lives within them, we are strengthened as a whole. As men and women stand side by side, we are a powerful force of love.

The Me Too Movement was important to bring truth to the surface. It also exposed a lot of anger. It is important not to hold onto the anger, but to give yourself permission to express it, release it, then go within it and draw out the wisdom within that. Anger is a natural human emotion. We do not want to repress it; we want to express it in a way that does not hurt another or ourselves. Then we must move through it, release it and rise up as a wiser self because of it.

The calling out had to happen. It had been suppressed for too long. Now that the calling out has taken place and as it continues to unfold, the important question to ask is, what will we now call forth? What will you call forth?

We are constantly redefining our roles as women and men. When we stand side by side, honor our differences, and express compassion for one another, leading with integrity, kindness, and respect, communities thrive.

Many men have become unsure of how to approach a woman. Companies and corporations fear the possibility of sexual harassment lawsuits. It's a confusing and frustrating time for many. This is one reason I am so passionate about teaching the art of mindful communication for couples, singles, and between men and women in the workplace. I have great faith that all is well and we're simply experiencing growing pains.

As adults we must teach by example and express self-love, honoring the beauty in ourselves and in one another, in all of our shapes, sizes, colors and age groups.

It is time to bring sex education out of the dark ages and include more conscious sex-ed in the schools. France is leading the way as a wonderful example, teaching a more conscious complete method of sex-ed, including the reality of pleasure in their teachings, and the fact that the clitoris exists, using a 3D model for their instruction.

The Netherlands is also a leader with sex education, with very low rates of teen age pregnancy through coherent sex-ed classes that include thorough teachings of safe sex. They also have a more advanced approach in their sex educational materials and in the classroom.

Our sexual expression shifts throughout the cycles in our lives for men and women. The youth are hungry for adults to teach the full spectrum of sexuality, not just on a physical technical level, but also emotionally and energetically.

CYCLES
"Honor your Body's Cycles.
The Moon Time of the Maiden and the Mother
brings cleansing and the possibility of new life.
The Completion of Moon Time in the Queen
and Sage brings new life to Sexual Expression.
There is vibrancy, radiance and
sacredness in all of life's stages.
Play with the blessing of this."
~ Sacred Sexual Enlightenment Wisdom Cards

I like to think of the male cycles as the Prince, the Enlightened Warrior, the King, and the Wisdom Keeper.

Whatever cycle you are in at this time, honor that in yourself and embrace the power and beauty of who you are. If you are mature, your wisdom is a gift to everyone who wishes to receive it. Just remember to recognize and listen to the wisdom of the youth as well.

I have great faith in our future. My young friends blow me away with their level of consciousness and wisdom. The new ones being born into this time do not enter into the consciousness we did at our point of entry. They are being born into the consciousness that exists now. Both the mature ones and the young ones are teachers we can all learn from.

CHAPTER 4

Sexual Evolution

"To me, if sex is the creative force in the world, it must be nearest to the creative center of the world— whatever name you give to it. Creative energy must be closest to creation, to the creative source of it all. People should be taught the art of converting sexual energy into spiritual enlightenment." ~ Osho

---

TANTRA & SACRED SEXUALITY

It seems no matter how often you ask for a definition of Tantra, you'll get a different answer. That's because it is too expansive to narrow it down to one answer. Tantra is a philosophy and way of life. Tantra is an ancient practice that originates from India. Its wisdom and practice have been around for thousands of years, passed down by various lineages. The Classic Tantriks of India are devoted to the ancient sacred texts, and primarily spiritual practices that include meditative practices, initiation, ritual, the worshiping of deities, and purification ceremonies. I have not yet been to India or studied under one of these lineages, so I can't speak about them in depth.

The Tantra practice most have become familiar with in the Western World is Neo-Tantra—the weaving together and exploration of spirituality and sexuality, also called Sacred Sexuality. I began the exploration of Neo-Tantra long before I had even heard of the word "Tantra," when my healing journey began in 1999. For me, the yearning to discover and explore my connection between God and my sexuality was a natural unfolding during this time. The practice and wisdom of Sacred Sexuality is my passion and the foundation of this book.

I am a guide and teacher of Neo-Tantra, I am also a student of Tantra and always will be. What I have learned up to now, I have learned from masters and through years of my own personal exploration.

A Tantric lifestyle encompasses all aspects of life, including how we explore our lives with family, how we treat other people, the Earth, all living things, and even our way of being in business. It is the magnification of polarities to where they become one... the Feminine and the Masculine, Spirituality and the Primal Physical, and so on. It is the exploration of polarities so fully that we take ourselves to the edge. As the polarities merge, higher states of consciousness and awakening take place.

Neo-Tantra and the ancient classic Tantra studies can differ greatly from one another; however, they share some common elements such as the weaving of the mind, physical body, soul and emotional body connection. Neo-Tantra and classic Tantra both integrate breath into their meditative practice and to transcend the state of being. I adore breath work. As a Certified Holistic Rebirther, breath plays a huge role in my healing practice, my meditation practice, and with sex. I have witnessed beautiful results in my clients through the teachings of Sacred Sexuality, combined with breath work and verbally guided techniques.

In Sanskrit, "tan" means "breath." You could say "Tantra" means "moving toward one's breath," or more clearly, "one's truth." The English word "tension" was derived from the word "Tantra." Imagine weaving two energies together, exploring the connection of these energies as far as possible, taking yourself to the edge without breaking the connection. Imagine the tension this creates. That is Tantra. The variations on how this can be applied are endless.

At a gathering in the home of my Vedic guru, Jeffrey Armstrong, the teaching he shared with us was spiritually and mentally stimulating. This is an example of non-sexual Tantra. The energy level in the room was raised so high that when it was time for a break, he requested that we remain silent. He knew that if we chattered, it would disrupt the energy and the tension would be broken. We could feel the beautiful tension linger in the air as we hurried back to our seats for more. He said to us, "Feel that tension as you hold onto the last moment and anticipant the next, that is Tantra."

Imagine you're at a concert and the music is exquisite. As you sing along, dance or simply listen, savoring the music, you can feel the vibration rising in the room. Imagine as one song completes, you feel the energy of it lingering in the air with the audience in silence. This silence between songs is common when attending a devotional music concert so as to not disperse the energy. During this silence, imagine feeling the tension as you anticipate the next song while still connected to the magic of the one just completed. That is Tantra.

Now imagine all the endless possibilities of exploring the connection between energies in all of existence. Imagine the possibilities as you explore and merge the polarities of Sexuality and Spirituality beyond your imagination. The journey is extraordinary and mind-blowing in relation to the new realms you experience of ecstatic pleasure while in union with God.

The chakras are the body's energy activation centers. Chakra is the Sanskrit word for "wheel," referring to the circular spinning shape of these energy centers. The activation of our upper chakras corresponds to our connection with the Divine realm, to our intuition and insight and our ability to speak our truth. Tantric practices that focus on these energies and our union with the Divine without the inclusion of sexuality is known as White Tantra.

The activation of our lower chakras corresponds to our connection with the physical primal realm, to our connection with the Earth, our survival, our sexual and creative energy as well as our emotional center and personal power. The heart chakra is at the center of this. As we explore the union of our Divine Spirit body with our primal Sexual body, this can only be done with an open heart and from a space of love. The heart is the core that makes this possible and the possibilities are endless.

SEXUAL EVOLUTION 53

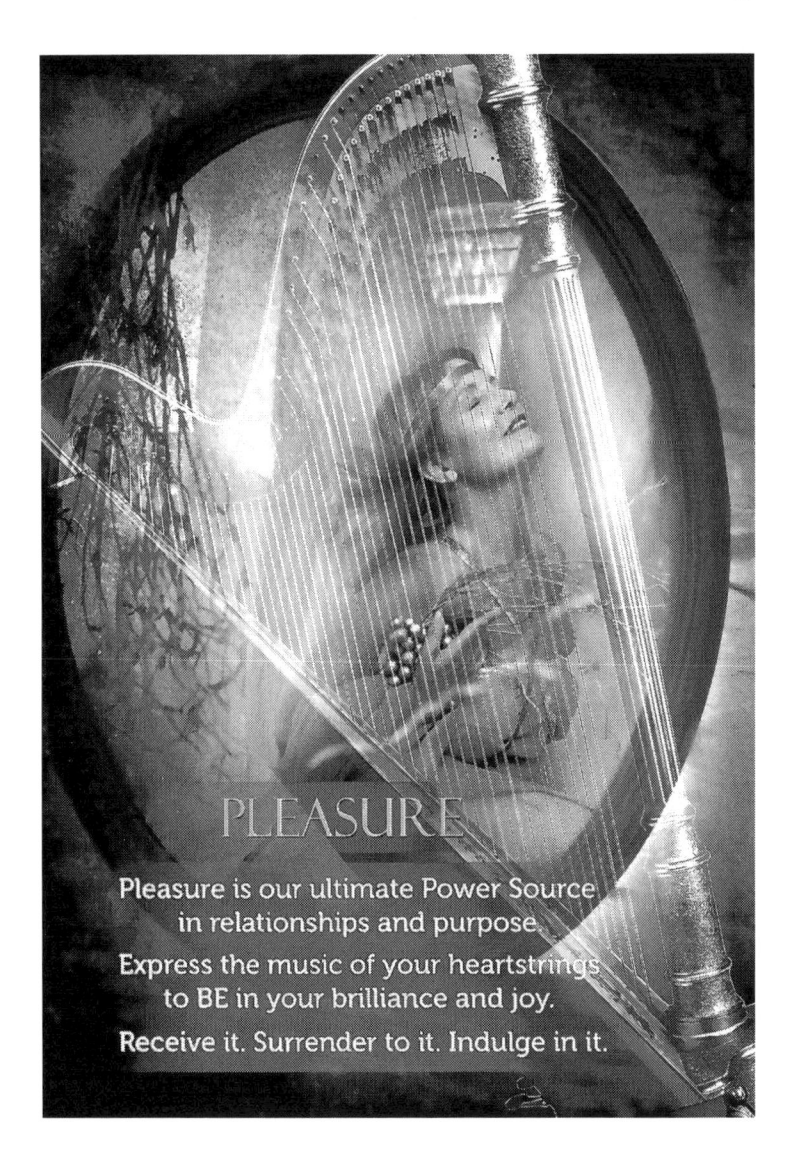

PLEASURE

Pleasure is our ultimate Power Source in relationships and purpose.

Express the music of your heartstrings to BE in your brilliance and joy.

Receive it. Surrender to it. Indulge in it.

To be Tantric is to be in full presence with self, the moment, and others; to be aware of the energy within you and around you; the energy you emanate and attract. A Tantric lifestyle is to be in awareness of the frequency you are generating in relation to what you receive back. It is awareness of how the energy you emanate impacts the unfolding of the next moment, and those around you. It is entering a knowing of who you are as the creator of your own reality, this dream called life, and your connection to Spirit and to all things. It is being in awareness of how you merge the energy of the masculine and feminine within you and with others. It is going to the edge and being in presence with various realms of possibility.

I've shared a few tidbits here with you. Diving into the depths of Tantra and all the realms of possibility is a devotion. We can never learn all there is to know about Tantra because it is a way of Being and an ongoing practice. It is ever unfolding, just like life. Even the teachers of Tantra are always students.

When we take responsibility for ourselves and are in full presence of our actions, our thoughts and daily interactions, our lives unfold with more grace. It is our nature as spiritual beings to be in a constant state of expansion and exploration.

If life appears to stagnate, you have probably forgotten who you are, caught up in the illusion that the physical plane is all that is. It is impossible to be stagnant. Life is always in a state of movement. We are either flourishing or deteriorating. Through conscious attention, you get to choose what direction you are going in. Why not choose the direction of expansion fueled by love, pleasure, peacefulness, and joy?

Sometimes those on a spiritual path may struggle with an either/or mindset, fearing that the desire to make money or placing importance on physicality will make them less spiritual. This is not an either/or situation. We came into this life as spiritual beings wanting a physical experience, with a desire to weave these two aspects of ourselves together and to explore life. Our sexuality is a beautiful aspect of this life. Explore it with an open heart. When you do this, the possibilities for inner peace and joy are endless. So, play with it!

LAYERS OF DISCOVERY

"Tantra is a totally different attitude. It says: There is joy in sex and there is frustration in sex. Because the moment of orgasm is very small.

That moment can become very deep, that moment can remain there for hours. That moment, once you know the art of remaining in it, can surround you twenty-four hours.

Tantra transforms sex. Tantra is the true religion.

It does not choose between the fascination and the frustration, it transcends both. It uses sex as a key.

And it is a key — because all life comes through it, all flowers bloom through it and all birds sing through it.

> *All that you see around you, the green and the red and the gold, all comes through sex and is sex energy.*
>
> *All the poetry and all the songs and all the music is rooted in sex-energy. All art, all creativity, is nothing but an expression of sex.*
>
> *So Tantra sex has to be understood.*
>
> *A few things: The Tantric definition of sexuality is opposite to the modern definition.*
>
> *The modern mind regards sex as a need – like hunger for food – which incidentally provides sense-and ego gratification. That's how Freud thinks about sex, that it gives you ego-gratification, satisfaction, relaxation; it relieves tensions, it is a need.*
>
> *Tantra regards sex as a powerful instinctual return to our ultimate reality, one of the highest forms of meditation."*
>
> ~ Osho

GOOD SEX IS a learned communicative skill. Great sex is an art form…giving, attentive, patient, soul to soul, intuitive, loving, playful, primal, healing and nurturing. Enlightened sex is all this and an ever-expanding weaving and merging of your physical body with your divinity.

We do not hit puberty and suddenly know what to do. During the early years of sexual expression, most are the blind leading the blind, with a basic understanding that the penis enters the vagina, left figuring out the rest through sex education that is very limited, or through books, porn, and personal exploration.

Many go well into adulthood still not understanding the full spectrum of what we are capable of sexually or how to show up as a good lover. Many will live their lives never knowing what it means to experience the full spectrum of ecstasy we are designed for; never understanding the freedom and beauty of who we are as both Divine and Sexual Beings.

The intention of this book is to remind you who you really are as a Divine Sexual Being. It is a guide to free yourself of past wounds and refill that space with wisdom, love, and lightness. It is a guide to experience healthier more joyful relationships, to live your ultimate love life with or without a partner, to enhance your creativity and this dream called life.

I can't provide you enlightenment. That's your journey. In this book I am giving you a guide, nudging you to explore aspects of your being in relation to the integral connection of your sexuality and your divinity. Enlightenment is not a destination. It is an ongoing journey of spiritual exploration, expansion, connection, and awakening.

Even if your path is celibacy, this book has great value for you. Sexual energy is your creative life force. The healthier it is, the more open the flow. You came from sex. You are a sexual being whether you're having sex or not. Sexual orgasmic energy gave you life and it infuses life and vitality within you.

We came into these bodies willingly and enthusiastically ready to savor the journey of discovery that life holds for us, for the sheer joy and exhilaration of it. We knew sexual expression would be a beautiful aspect of this journey called life. We came here with full awareness that sexual expression is a precious Divine gift of life, pleasure, healing, connection, joy and bliss. Do you feel the truth of these words in your soul?

Be in the joy of this dance of sexual discovery and evolution. Stay open to all the possibilities of healing, exploration, surrender, love, joy, expansion, expression, and awakened ecstasy... with or without a partner.

Part Two

The Four Sacred Laws *of* Sexual Enlightenment

CHAPTER 5

The Gift

The 1st Sacred Law of Sexual Enlightenment is **THE GIFT**
—Honoring sexual energy as a multidimensional Gift.

CREATION
"You're a Sacred Being inside a Sacred Body.
Sexual Energy is the Power Cord connecting the
transcendental realm to the physical realm.
Embrace the beauty and wholeness of this."
~ *Sacred Sexual Enlightenment Wisdom Cards*

SEX CREATES our existence as a Divine Being having this physical human experience. Sexuality is not intended to be an expression separate from God. It is an expression of God. When the orgasmic body merges with the Divine Spirit body, the pleasure is most potent.

This is our Divine Design.

THE GIFT OF LIFE

Your father had an orgasm which planted the seed that created your existence as a spiritual being in a physical body. Ideally, your mother was also orgasmic at your time of conception. Either way, sex and orgasm are responsible for your physical existence and the Gift of life in your body.

We activate our sexual energy to create the Gift of human life. We also activate sexual energy for the Gift of pleasure and to breathe new life through us. If sexual energy were only intended for procreation, then women would only ovulate every nine months, just as a dog only goes into heat every six months. Our bodies are intentional miracles of creation. Creation intended for us to experience pleasure through sexual activation whenever we choose. It is our Divine Design, or it would not be possible.

When we embrace sexual energy as a sacred Gift, then we honor it, respect it and cherish it, just as we would honor, respect, and cherish any Gift we receive with unconditional love. With this honoring, we can eliminate the judgment, constriction, repression, anxiety or shame that is often connected with sexuality. We become more protective of our sexual energy just as we would be protective of any Gift we receive from someone special in our lives. By protective I mean we are more discerning about who we share our precious and powerful sexual life force energy with.

When we acknowledge that sexual energy is a Gift and embrace this as truth, we do not put it in a separate category from who we are spiritually. The taboo of it slips away and instead, we reclaim our powerful truth of who we are as sacred beings in these sacred physical primal orgasmic bodies.

THE BODY TEMPLE

> *"The body is so loyal, even when we judge it or hurt it. We need to honor our temple, be gentle and generous with our temple. No one can be as generous with our temple as much as we can. Never allow anybody including yourself to disrespect your temple."*
> ~ *Don Miguel Ruiz; Circle of Fire Gathering 2018*

YOUR BODY IS A TEMPLE… a miracle… a Gift created for pleasure. Every single part of our body is as Sacred as any another. Our genitals are as Sacred as our eyes. Our rectum is as sacred as our hands, and so on. Every part of us is designed perfectly, serves a specific purpose and contributes to the quality and pleasure of life in a physical body. It really is a miracle. Our sexual energy and sexual reproductive systems create the miracle of life in this physical realm. What a Gift!

There is an abundance of words used to name our genitalia. I found a webpage listing 159 words for women alone. Some were pleasant, some crude and some humorous. Vagina is limiting, as it is the medical word for the muscular canal extending from the cervix to the outside of the body. It does not include the clitoris, vulva or labia. Pussy is quite common, but still limiting, referring to the exterior genitalia and vagina but not typically including the uterus or womb. I love the Sanskrit word "yoni." I've heard some say they find this word pretentious. I disagree.

I love "yoni" because it is all encompassing, representing all parts of a woman's sexual anatomy as well as its essence. In Sanskrit yoni is defined as vagina, vulva, uterus, womb, a symbol of Divine procreative energy, place of birth, origin, source, place of rest, abode, home and nest. Yoni is also spring and fountain, acknowledging the messiness and beauty of nectar flowing through arousal. The word for clitoris is, "YoniliGga," and acknowledged as an aspect of the yoni. Yoni is a symbol of the Goddess, or Shakti, female creative energy. It is seen as nature's gateway to all births... a portal.

I searched but I could not find an article with one or two names that men preferred over others for penis. Commonly used words varied with nationality. I read about a study done on men in their twenties and none of the common words appealed to them, as they did not like their penis separated from who they are as a man. I love that. When I am with a lover, I will say, "I want you inside me," versus, "I want your penis inside me."

When a lover says, "I want to be inside you," verses " I want to be inside your pussy," it creates deeper connection. When in the throes of passion, by not separating genitals from the person, we integrate the body temple in all its beauty and messiness with the soul of the person we are with.

YONI

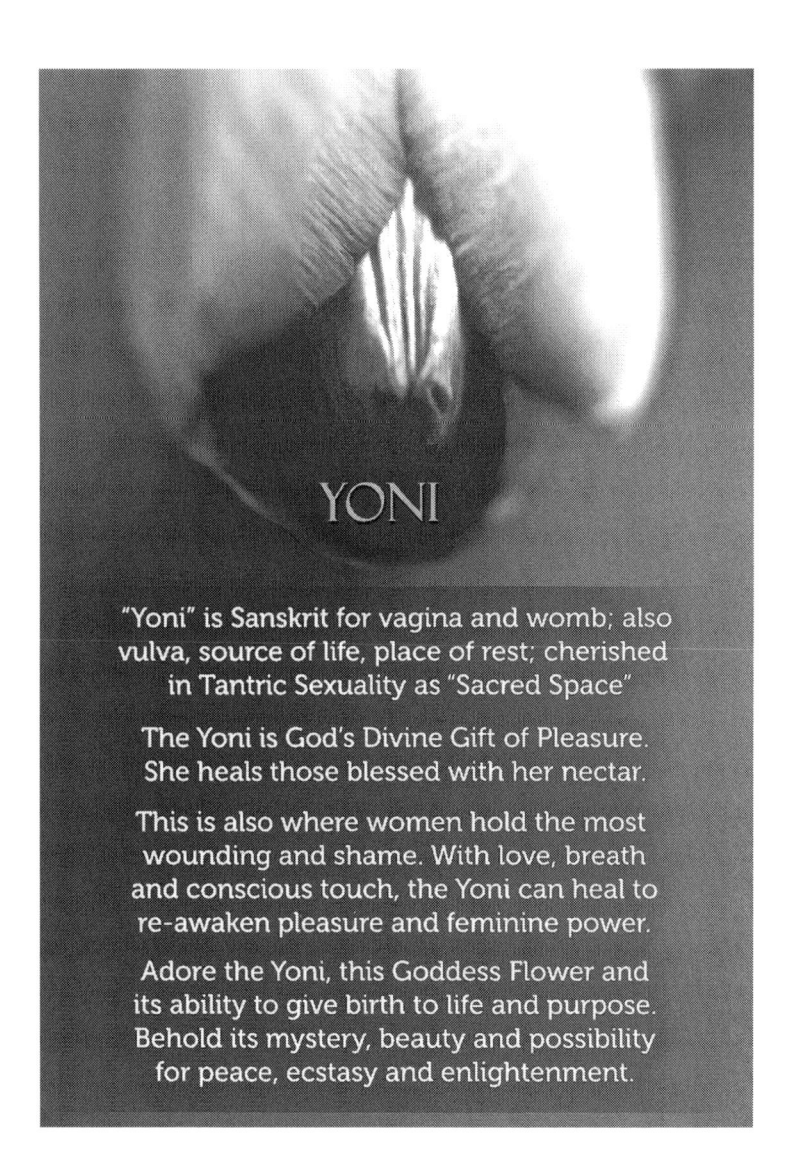

"Yoni" is Sanskrit for vagina and womb; also vulva, source of life, place of rest; cherished in Tantric Sexuality as "Sacred Space"

The Yoni is God's Divine Gift of Pleasure. She heals those blessed with her nectar.

This is also where women hold the most wounding and shame. With love, breath and conscious touch, the Yoni can heal to re-awaken pleasure and feminine power.

Adore the Yoni, this Goddess Flower and its ability to give birth to life and purpose. Behold its mystery, beauty and possibility for peace, ecstasy and enlightenment.

LINGAM

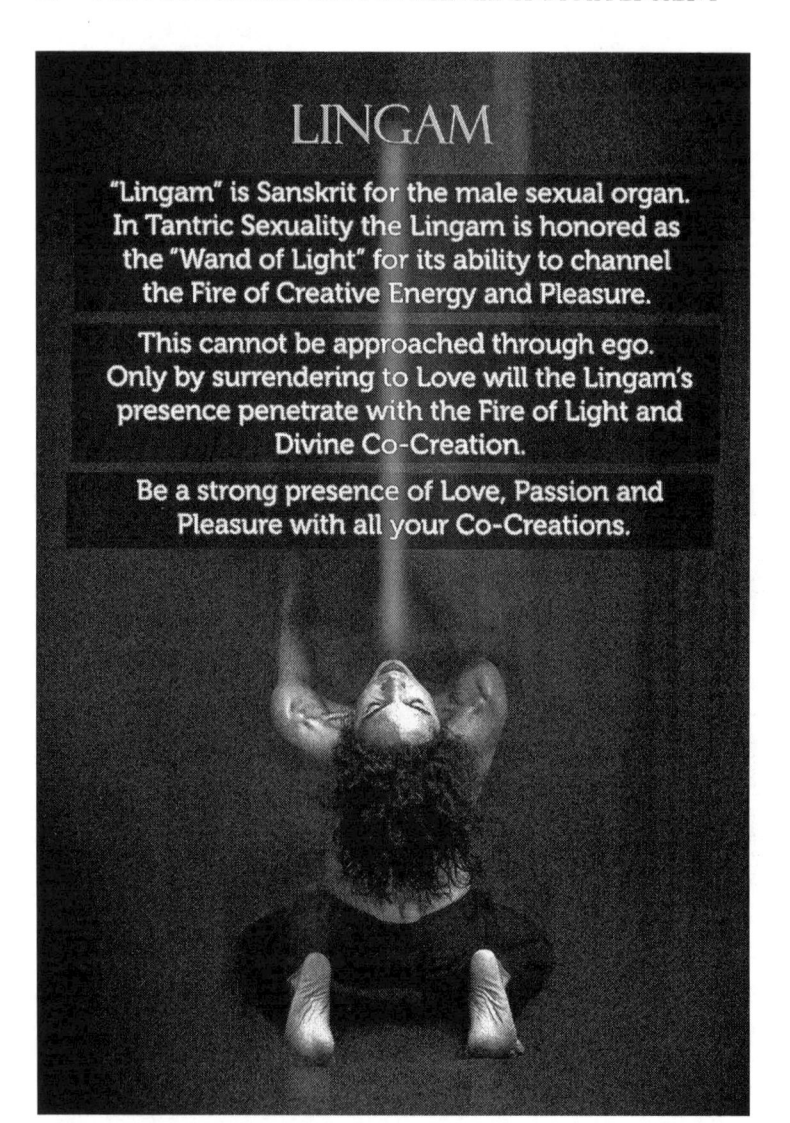

"Lingam" is Sanskrit for the male sexual organ. In Tantric Sexuality the Lingam is honored as the "Wand of Light" for its ability to channel the Fire of Creative Energy and Pleasure.

This cannot be approached through ego. Only by surrendering to Love will the Lingam's presence penetrate with the Fire of Light and Divine Co-Creation.

Be a strong presence of Love, Passion and Pleasure with all your Co-Creations.

"Lingam" also known as "linga" is the Sanskrit word for penis and has diverse meanings. Some of these are, mark, sign, token, badge, emblem, symbol and proof. Lingam means image of God, idol, male organ or phallus, beginning-less and endless cosmic pillar of fire. It is a symbol of the God Shiva who protects, creates and transforms the universe. The lingam is recognized as a wand of light when shared with conscious connection and love.

Yoni is honored as sacred for her powers of creation, birth and mystery. The lingam is honored as sacred and a potent phallic current of life force energy merging a man's body with divinity.

As a man enters a woman, her yoni is a portal to union with the Divine Feminine. As the woman receives him inside her, the lingam is a current filling her with Divine Masculine connection. As we bring our beautiful body temples together connecting heart to heart, soul to soul, we merge with God within and beyond. Is it any wonder when in orgasmic bliss, our nature is to call out, "Oh God!"

You get to name your genitals whatever you want. I recommend choosing one that honors your body as the temple it is. Make up your own if you want to. Your body is intelligent. Words carry frequencies. Try tuning into your body and ask your yoni or lingam what name resonates and see what comes to you, and choose what feels good to you.

MULTIPLE DIMENSIONS OF THE GIFT

Imagine you craft the most beautiful exquisite Gift and you give it to someone who you love dearly. Imagine this person is a musician. Imagine this Gift is a musical instrument and you pour all of your heart and soul into making sure that this Gift is designed perfectly in every detail. Imagine you then present this to the person you love. Imagine this Gift has twelve strings on it, and although they receive the Gift and they appreciate it, they only play one or two strings.

The instrument may still sound very beautiful playing one or two strings, however, are they fully honoring the Gift as it was intended? If instead, they learn how to play the instrument with all twelve strings, they have a more beautiful, fulfilling, multi-dimensional experience with their musical Gift, as do those who receive their Gift by sharing it with them.

What about you? Are you honoring the Gift of sexuality as Creation intended, or are you just playing one or two strings... only expressing one or two layers? Are you exploring all the layers the Gift of your sexual energy has to offer you?

What if you gave someone a precious Gift and they judged it somehow? That does not feel in alignment, does it? Our sexual energy is no different. Our sexual energy is a Gift that is an integral aspect of our Divine Creation. As emotional wounding, shame or judgment is cleared one can move from feeling contraction into feeling expansive and step into all the power, sacredness, beauty and dimensions of *The Gift*.

The Second Chakra, known in Sanskrit as the

Svadhisthana, and also called the Sacral Chakra, is the energy activation center for our creative energy as well as the activation center for pleasure and sexual energy. They are one and the same. We are created through orgasmic sexual energy, so our sexual energy is literally at the root source of our creative expression.

Even if you don't consider yourself a creative person, the fact is you are creating your own life. Your life is your art.

If the energy of your Sacral Chakra is blocked, it can show up in your life as feelings of insecurity, lack of self-confidence, difficulty keeping your emotions in balance and difficulty associating with other people and the world around you. When your Sacral Chakra is activated, it opens you to feel passionate, sensual, creatively inspired, emotionally stable, connected and joyful. You will also feel very present in your body.

Whenever there is judgment, guilt, confusion, wounding, or disconnect within the sexual energy, the Sacral Chakra becomes blocked and closed off. This results in a holding back to protect this vulnerable aspect of self. When you're holding back you're holding back... period.

When the roots of a tree are constricted, it stunts the entire tree's growth and it can never blossom to its full potential. With sexual energy being the root of our creation, this holding back stunts the layers of your expression; what you create in relationships, and everything else in life.

So, can you be celibate and still be in the full power of your creativity? Absolutely! But, only if this is a choice made through inner peace and contentment. Choosing a path of celibacy out of avoidance due to wounding, fear or contraction is disempowering and blocks creativity. As you free yourself from the energy charge at the Source of your wounds and contraction, the fullness of your personal and creative expression will open.

The more you open to the multidimensionality of your sexual life force energy, the more you open to possibility with love and in the creation of your life as a magnificent work of art. The more you embrace *The Gift* in all its layers, the more depth you feel in sexual intimacy with or without a partner.

Observe the orchid flower. It is the most honored, precious, valuable flower on the planet. It must be treated with great care, respect and delicacy for it to blossom. It is also very durable… just like the sex of a woman.

I believe the orchid was intentionally created to resemble the sex of a woman as a message from God saying, "Look precious woman, this is you! This is how you are to see yourself as this beautiful, beautiful flower."

Think about it… the clitoris has 6,000 to 8,000 nerve endings and is the only human body part created for the sole purpose of pleasure. What an incredible Gift and such a powerful message that women thrive through pleasure.

A woman's clitoris is more mysterious to a man than the penis is to a woman. I have had young men come to me as clients who didn't understand where the clitoris even was or how to stimulate it. This is true of the g-spot as well.

Giving sexual pleasure artfully to a man requires education, practice, and communication. Giving sexual pleasure artfully to a woman requires education, practice, and communication. It also requires patience and heart connection.

YOUR FLOWER

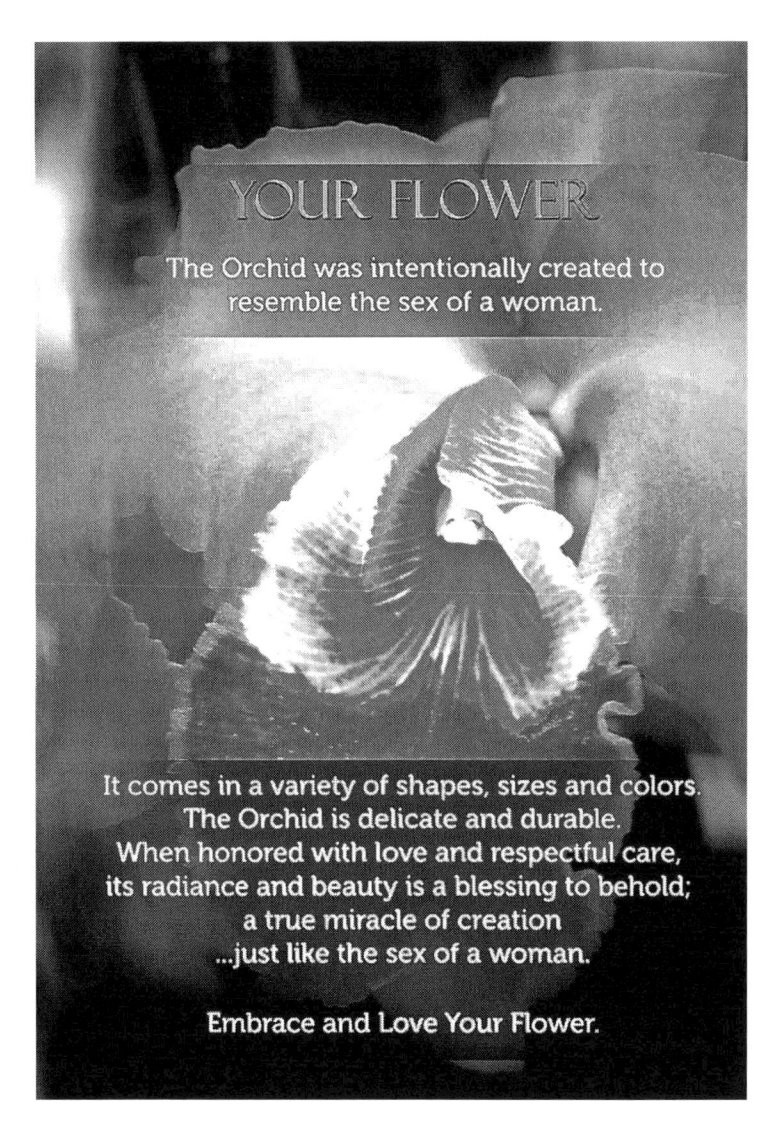

The Orchid was intentionally created to resemble the sex of a woman.

It comes in a variety of shapes, sizes and colors.
The Orchid is delicate and durable.
When honored with love and respectful care,
its radiance and beauty is a blessing to behold;
a true miracle of creation
...just like the sex of a woman.

Embrace and Love Your Flower.

An artist does not just slap something together and call it art. A true artist takes their time, draws from inspiration, attentive to their canvas and the creativity flowing through them, connecting fully as they give to their art.

The connection of your heart to your sex happens naturally when it's with someone you share a deep love with. You can also share this connection with a one-time encounter, or short-term relationship. Take the time and energy to look into the eyes of the one who has chosen to share their body with you and see the beauty that is them, honoring them and feeling the love that exists within them. Do this before you have sex with them.

When you penetrate their heart and their soul first, the beauty of the experience is magnified. Why discount connecting in this way just because you know it is temporary no matter how short? You're there anyway, so show up fully. To do otherwise is to cheat yourself and them of *The Gift* and what is possible at the moment.

Heart connection with sex can also take place without a partner. My solo practice integrates my sexual energy with my love of self and my connection to Source. When I'm single, I'm mostly celibate, yet my sex life is sacred, heart opening and ecstatic. It is fulfilling physically, emotionally and spiritually. To be with another, they must be able to meet me there, otherwise it feels incomplete. I share more with you on how to be in this sacred self-pleasure in the Chapter, *The Invitation*.

For some of you reading this, you may believe masturbation is a low form of sexual expression. You may have even been scolded as a child and made to feel shameful when touching yourself. I want to absolve you of this myth right now. Think about it; being told that it is bad to touch your own genitals is like saying that someone who you probably haven't met yet has more of a right to touch your own body than you do.

Your body is a Sacred Gift to you. You have more of a right to touch it than anyone. When you share it with another, you are sharing a precious Gift with them. God does not judge you for wanting to adore and enjoy pleasure with the Gift of your own body. You are the love of your life. Treat yourself as such. Touch yourself with all of the love you have inside you.

When you choose to share your body with another, they are a reflection of your self-love. If you don't like the reflection that is showing up, turn within. Observe how you can honor the love of your life more… you. Then you will attract that love in another.

Masturbation only risks being a sexual addiction when it is solely based on the physical release, void of emotional and spiritual integration. Experiencing physical release on its own can feel good physically, but if it becomes compulsive, then yes, there is a problem. It is also very one-dimensional.

Self-pleasure teaches you about your own body and how you want to be touched, so you can better guide your partner. Self-pleasure that expresses self-love and integrates spiritual connection is more expansive and multi-dimensional. When a partner makes this emotional and spiritual connection with you, the experience is magnified even more. It is a Union of extraordinary bliss.

DANCE OF MASCULINE & FEMININE

Delight in the dance of the Masculine and Feminine and the Gift of this within self and with others.

In this book, I refer to the Masculine and Feminine often. When I do so, I am not necessarily referring to men or women. I am referring to the Masculine and Feminine sexual essence that exists in each of us, regardless of sexual orientation or gender.

Most men have more of a Masculine sexual essence. Most women have more of a Feminine sexual essence. The degrees vary. A woman can have more of a Masculine essence and a man more of a Feminine. There are some who are neutral. You probably have a good sense of what your primary sexual essence is. So, from this point forward, as I speak into the Masculine and Feminine, relate to that aspect of yourself. If you're in a relationship, relate to that aspect of your partner as well.

Aspects of Masculine essence are consciousness and physical. Aspects of Feminine essence are spiritual and emotional. The Feminine gets sexually aroused through emotional stimulation. The Masculine gets emotionally stimulated from physical arousal. I know this may seem like a cosmic joke, but when you understand the nuances of the dance of Masculine and Feminine, it is a never-ending flow of intriguing exploration.

In the teachings of my friend and mentor, Satyen Raja, I love how beautifully he shares that when one is strong in their Masculine, they have the qualities of presence, claim and penetration. When one is strong in their Feminine, they have the qualities of invitation, surrender and expression.

So, in this section on the *Dance of Masculine and Feminine*, as I use the language of Masculine presence, claim and penetration and how that merges with Feminine invitation, surrender and expression, I am integrating Satyen's teachings with mine, and am grateful and honored for his permission to do so.

The Feminine is emotionally driven to sex with the Masculine, which opens and activates her to engage and express more physically. The Masculine is physically driven to sex with the Feminine, which opens and activates him to engage and express more emotionally. We are each Feminine and Masculine, primal and spiritual. The Feminine is flowing, nurturing, sensual. The Masculine is logical, protective, focused. Explore and express all aspects and polarities.

Do not buy into the myth that men just want sex and women just want connection. We both want both. We simply have unique perspectives. Women want ecstatic sexual pleasure while experiencing deep connection with their partner. Men want deep connection while witnessing ecstatic pleasure in their partner.

Both men and women desire fulfillment on all levels... emotionally, spiritually, mentally and physically. Our unique perspectives as Masculine and Feminine are part of the dance, and it's so beautiful when we embrace that and are in rhythm with one another.

When the adolescent Masculine is focused on physically penetrating the Feminine, he resembles a panting puppy. The mature Masculine knows to look into her eyes and penetrate her heart and soul first. When she feels this connection deep in her core, it inspires her to invite him in.

She doesn't feel the need to be in love with him to extend an invitation, but she does want to feel safe in his presence, to feel a connection and to feel her heart center open. A woman's, heart and yoni are energetically connected.

When a woman decides to have sex without feeling emotionally stimulated by some kind of a heart connection to her sexual partner, it's likely due to one of the following:

- Her Masculine essence is more dominant.
- Physical sex void of heart connection has been her only experience, and although she likely desires more, she has sex as a misaligned way to try and achieve connection.
- She is at a time where raw primal sex on its own is a temporary fix to relieve pent up energy.
- She has a protective shield around her heart due to unresolved emotional wounding, so she cannot fully surrender, open and receive the sexual experience in all its elements of body, heart, soul connection.

When a woman has a more of a Feminine essence, it is natural to respond to the Masculine's lead the majority of the time. This is true with dancers on the dance floor and in the dance of relationships. However, the woman who is more Feminine may still want to initiate sex occasionally, in fact, I recommend it. To do this, it means she must activate that aspect of her that is Masculine and he must surrender to the aspect of himself that is Feminine. This does not mean he acts effeminate. It simply means he surrenders to her invitation and initiation.

YONI HEART

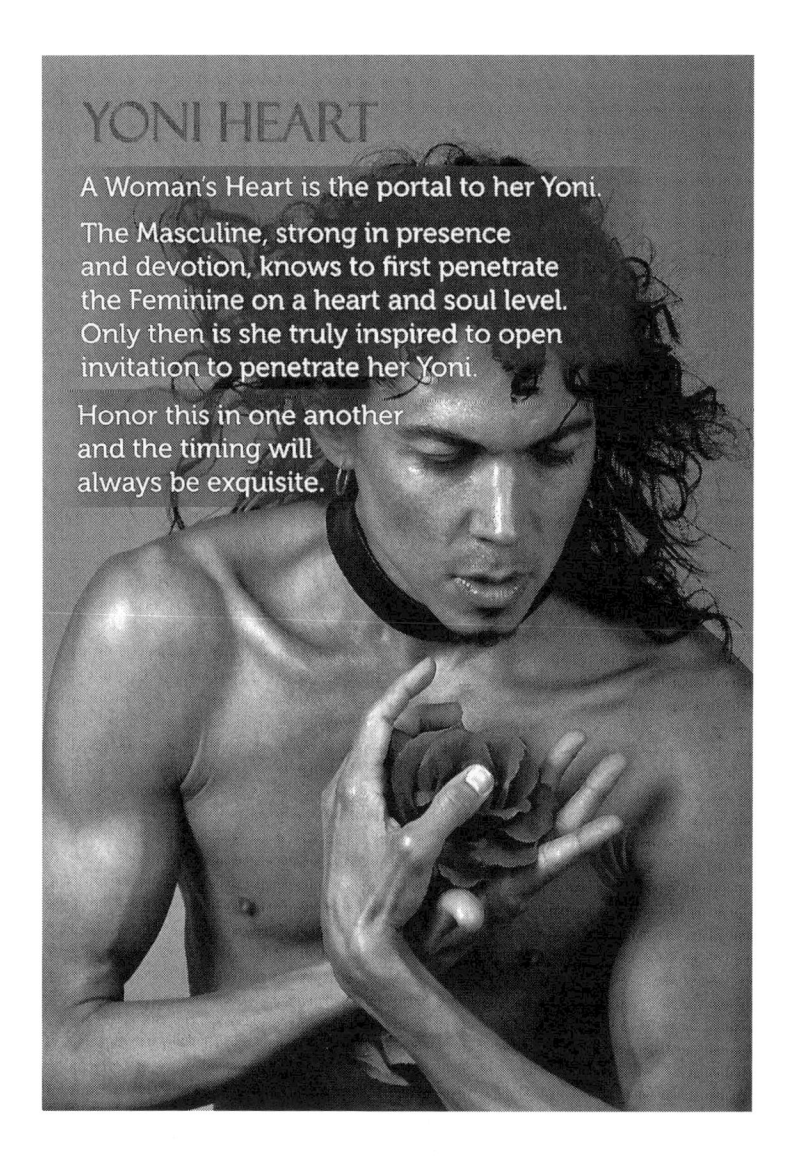

A Woman's Heart is the portal to her Yoni.

The Masculine, strong in presence and devotion, knows to first penetrate the Feminine on a heart and soul level. Only then is she truly inspired to open invitation to penetrate her Yoni.

Honor this in one another and the timing will always be exquisite.

In the chapter, *History and Herstory* I shared how the Priestesses of ancient temples would nurture the war out of the warriors with their healing gifts of Sacred Sexuality. Women, be aware of the weary warrior. No man is 100% Masculine essence and you would not want him to be. It's exhausting to hold strong in this presence all the time. At times he needs to be able to surrender and have his Feminine counterpart stand in her presence and hold space for him so he can let go and recharge.

When a woman takes care of business, whether at the office or as a stay at home mom, she must be more in her Masculine essence. She's making decisions, in control, and getting the job done. She's in warrior mode. If she stays there when with her man, the polarities will not match up for intimacy to spark. Men, you can help her by taking over parenting responsibilities while she has a bath, or by giving her a foot massage; whatever it takes, so she can let go and relax back into what is the natural state of Feminine essence for her.

It's so sexy when a woman feels trust, safe to surrender and says to her man through her words or body language, "just take me!" It is so sexy when a man responds and is powerful in his passion for her and claims her. This is not surrender in the sense of giving up or as in submission. This is about surrendering while in the power of her radiance. When these agreements are in place, it is a huge turn on for both.

As the Feminine, how are you inviting the Masculine in? It can be as simple as, "Come sit with me." Or an inviting smile welcoming him toward you. If you are not inviting, why would he want to be present with you? Open to him, inviting him into your space, inviting him in to come closer to you.

The motivating force behind a woman's existence is love: giving love, receiving love, feeling deeply loved, and experiencing love. The Feminine aspect of a woman will either open in loving surrender or close through a sense of protection. The motivating force to a man's existence is freedom. Yes, love for him is a priority as well, but freedom more so. A man must feel free to hold on to his vision and pursue it, or he weakens and cheats his woman of his authentic self.

A man strong in presence is very alluring and attractive. If you are the Masculine, answer these questions: what do you stand for? Who do you love? What is your purpose? What is your mission? If you don't know, figure it out. You will feel more aligned and empowered and be more attractive to the Feminine.

When the Masculine carries the energy of "I am with you. I am beside you. I am behind you. Let's go here..." That is very sexy to the Feminine.

To be strong in presence, a man must show up in purpose, his mission and dedication. To know what he is a stand for and claim it. When a man lacks presence it weakens the sexual attraction. In relationships, it can show up as the Feminine going more into her Masculine to compensate.

Years ago, I lived with a man for three years whose presence was weak and didn't really take a stand for anything. His presence and passion was strong in the bedroom and was a giving lover, but outside of the bedroom he did not stand powerfully in his Masculine. He still carried wounds from the ongoing criticism of his father. He didn't have a mission in life and would not make decisions about things as simple as where to go on our night out. Though I loved him deeply, this aspect of him was a turn off for me.

I ended up being the decision maker in the relationship. I didn't want to be in control all the time, but because I was less evolved, I reacted by becoming controlling. He and I did not have this knowledge back then, or the communication skills to shift our relationship, so it ended. I wasn't aware that I was longing for him to step more fully into the power of his Masculine and to claim me and his love for me, so I could more fully surrender. The Gift of this relationship is the love that remains and the wisdom the lessons brought me.

The Feminine is the receptor. The Masculine is the penetrator. Just look at our physical bodies; it's obvious. A woman's sex extends inside her body. A man's sex extends outside his body. The Feminine's nature is to respond to what she is receiving. The Masculine's nature is to move forward… to penetrate.

DIVINE MASCULINE

"The Divine Masculine provides safety, witnesses without judgment and holds space. Be this, and you are her King.
A Feminine in self-judgment, disconnects from him within, does not feel safe and holds back.
Goddess, align with your inner Divine Masculine, and feel safe to let go, surrender and fully express."
~ Sacred Sexual Enlightenment Wisdom Cards

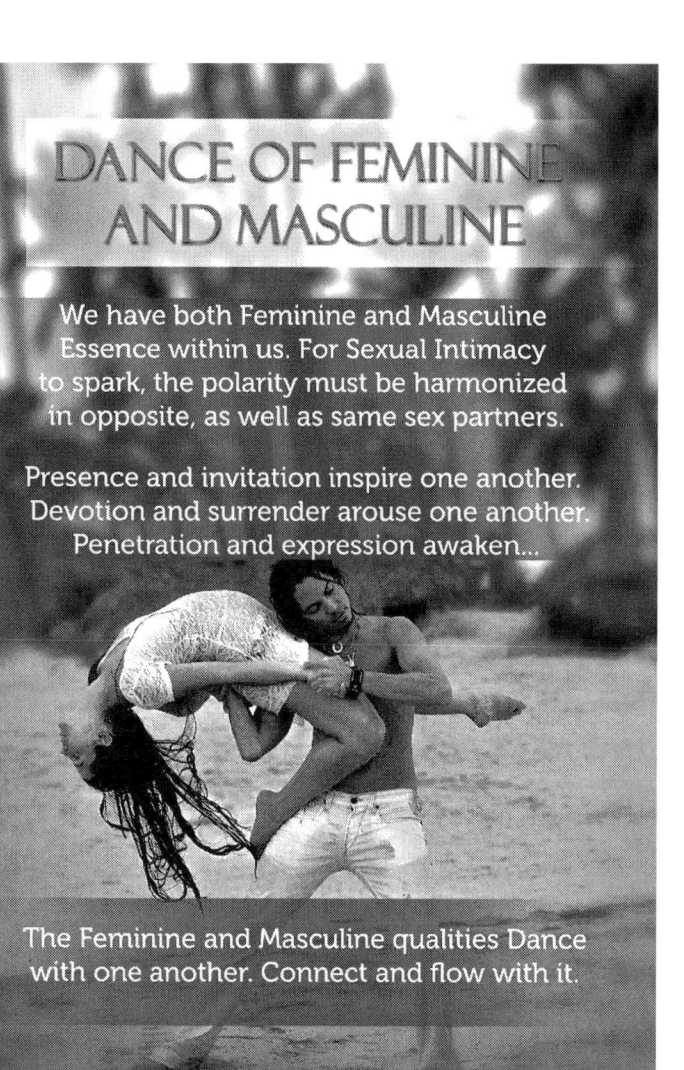

DANCE OF FEMININE AND MASCULINE

We have both Feminine and Masculine Essence within us. For Sexual Intimacy to spark, the polarity must be harmonized in opposite, as well as same sex partners.

Presence and invitation inspire one another. Devotion and surrender arouse one another. Penetration and expression awaken...

The Feminine and Masculine qualities Dance with one another. Connect and flow with it.

DIVINE FEMININE
"The Divine Feminine is love, nurturing, and compassion.
She cannot be rushed to primal touch.
She requires connection, tenderness,
and an intuitive touch tuned into her breath.
A Masculine who penetrates her soul, savors and opens
her slowly, is blessed with the splendor of drinking
in all her Wild Love, Fierceness and Divine Nectar.
Align with her, your inner Divine Feminine
to find strength in gentleness.
Love is her power."
~ Sacred Sexual Enlightenment Wisdom Cards

ONE INSPIRES THE OTHER...

When a Masculine is strong in presence offering his full attention, he inspires the Feminine to extend invitation. The more she extends her invitation, the more she inspires him to be in his presence and maintain it.

As the Masculine stands powerfully in his desire, claiming his devotion to his Feminine lover, the safer she feels and the more aroused she becomes, opening in trust, surrender and devotion to him. The more she trusts and surrenders in arousal, the more she inspires him to step up and move forward in his devotion and purpose.

As the Masculine penetrates the heart and soul of his beloved, feeling her inner truth, the more the deliciousness of her Feminine expression is awakened; more and more inviting him in; more and more opening to the fullness of her pleasure and expression. This in turn, awakens the truth of divine union within him, inspiring him to more deeply penetrate the soul of her being.

ARE you not receiving the intimacy or passion you desire in a relationship? Be the one to initiate the dance.

Are you the Feminine? Invite him in with your radiant smile. Offer your man your trust. Surrender to the passion he longs to give you. Give him the Gift of your expression. Move your body, laugh, giggle, growl, moan in delight, roar, express! Express tenderly and express your wild primal self.

Are you the Masculine? Give her your full, undivided presence and attention. Stand powerfully in your desire and devotion. Claim it. Penetrate deep into the core of her heart and soul. Then, behold the glorious divine union as together you bask in the ecstasy of body penetration.

"The way a man penetrates the world should be the same way he penetrates his woman: not merely for personal gain or pleasure, but to magnify love, openness, and depth."
~David Deida

LEARNING to master the dance of your inner Masculine and Feminine in yourself and with your partner is a beautiful aspect of the Gift. I love exploring this dance with my clients in our private couple's sessions and in my workshops. It never ceases to fascinate me how the polarities play themselves out.

Couples can experience a variety of issues that result in a disconnect with their sex life such as stress, money issues, over worked, health, or unhealthy patterns. I've chosen to bring attention to the following two:

1. The Feminine Is Too Mothering. When a woman is too mothering, she can repel her man. It creates a mother/son dynamic that is not sexy. An example is, a woman telling her man how to do household chores as she would speak to a son. This is emasculating. Do not allow your partnership to take on a parent/child dynamic. You are lovers.

Acts of service is one of the 5 Love Languages. If you are not familiar with these, go take the quiz at 5LoveLanguages.com. If it is a turn on for you when your partner contributes acts of service, then communicate that it's a turn on, versus ordering them about. Your Love Language is what you intuitively give to the other because it's what you want to receive. If their Love Language is different, they will give you that instead, and then you are a mismatch. Take the quiz and give the Love Language each wants to receive to one another.

The Feminine is naturally nurturing. Motherly nurturing may feel good, but no healthy man wants to have sex with his mother. Motherly nurturing does not invite sexual intimacy; it blocks it. Nurture your Beloved as the lover, not the mother.

2. The Masculine Not Taking Enough Time. The Masculine is goal oriented. So, when he becomes familiar with his partner's body and knows how to bring her to orgasm, he may have a tendency to touch and enter the yoni too soon. He may fall into the habit of leaving out the stimulation of words, eye contact, touch and kisses on the other parts of the body that caress and open her heart center. I hear this often from women who have been in a relationship with the same man for a long time. This can also show up with new lovers if the man is inexperienced, or unaware.

The Masculine may believe that if his partner has had an orgasm, she's had a good time. The orgasm feels good, but without taking the time to establish a heart arousal connection and extended foreplay, to her sex feels incomplete, yet she may stay silent and not share this with him. Many women struggle with communication around sex, more so than men. When a woman doesn't speak up and communicate her lack of fulfillment, it's usually because she wants him to feel like a good lover and not hurt his feelings, even when her desire does not match her experience.

Foreplay can begin at the breakfast table with a sexy note next to the coffee cup, or a soft caress and kiss on the neck before going to work, followed by tempting texts throughout the day, or a sexy phone call. Then, when together again, taking time to caress her face, her shoulders, legs and making eye contact connection.

He can take his time, exploring her entire body, holding off on touching her yoni until the anticipation is so high that she is moist and wet with arousal, relaxed and swelling, emotionally and physically prepared for penetration. The longer a man takes his time, building the anticipation, the more potent the pleasure will be for the woman when he penetrates her yoni, and the healthier it will be for her body.

Rushed intercourse can damage ligaments at the entrance of the vagina, which in turn can also damage the bladder and rectum. I share more in Chapter 8 in the subchapter, *Responsibility of Body Awareness*.

Maybe through lack of experience, knowledge or an emotional block, a woman has trouble reaching orgasm so she fakes it with the intention of protecting her partner's ego. Or maybe she convinces him that having an orgasm is not important to her because her heart feels full. Maybe through lack of control, the man reaches orgasm before the woman reaches hers.

Do you recognize yourself in any of these scenarios? These are common issues that many couples fall into. As it continues, she will feel more like she is servicing him, versus responding to him. A woman's love for her Beloved may hold her there, but she may eventually lose interest in having sex with him altogether. Most men want to be the hero for his woman. Both partners must communicate openly and honestly.

Most premature ejaculation issues can be easily resolved by learning to work with the breath and PC muscles. When a couple I'm working with has this problem, the first thing I discover is if the source of the problem is an emotional issue. If so, we address that first and clear the emotions that are the root of the problem. The good news is, something can be done about it.

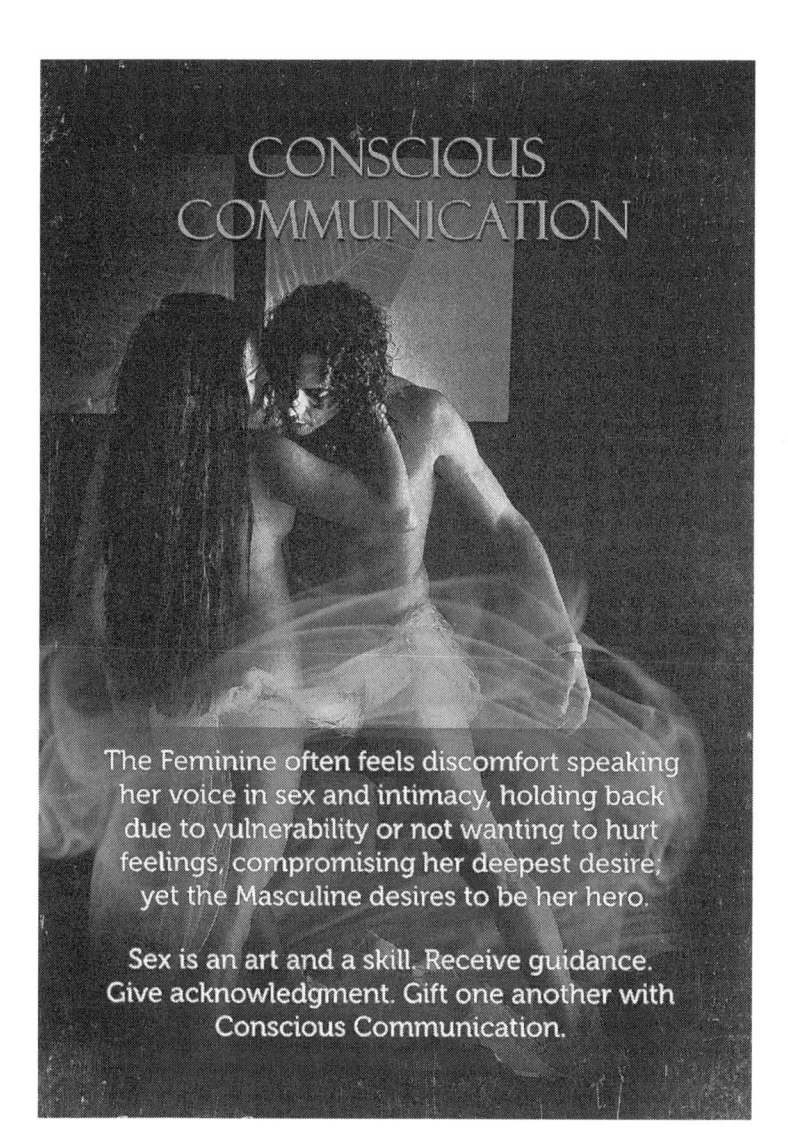

CONSCIOUS COMMUNICATION

The Feminine often feels discomfort speaking her voice in sex and intimacy, holding back due to vulnerability or not wanting to hurt feelings, compromising her deepest desire, yet the Masculine desires to be her hero.

Sex is an art and a skill. Receive guidance. Give acknowledgment. Gift one another with Conscious Communication.

If a partner is shy about asking for what they want sexually, encourage them by asking questions. See one another's bodies as a canvas of discovery. To explore the art of Sacred Sexuality, you must slow down... really slow down. Our bodies are miracles that house our soul... a Gift of creation. Take time to honor that.

Acknowledge what is good about your sex life. Share what you want more of or what you want to try. Be one another's guide and be playful with it.

When another shares their body with you, they are giving you a precious Gift. Be fully present with one another. Connect. Gaze deep into one another's eyes and see the soul of this beautiful one offering themselves to you. Feel one another's breath. Explore them slowly, breathing in every beautiful aspect of their Being.

Touch one another's body from a place of awe and wonder each and every time, as though you are seeing them for the very first time, even when you have been with them for years.

Even though women are designed to receive, it is the art of receiving that many women need help and support with. When a man truly takes his time, he helps her and supports her to relax, open and receive. When the man excels in the joy of giving her pleasure and has filled her up first, emotionally, spiritually and physically, she finds it easier to relax and open to receive.

As a woman opens to receive what her partner is giving her, then she also opens to receiving more pleasure in the giving. What a Gift it is for the Masculine when the Feminine fully indulges in receiving pleasure from the giving of pleasure.

When I guide couples in the art of giving a sensual massage to one another, often the Masculine partner feels the need to be "doing." This often translates into his hands moving quickly over her body so he feels like he is moving forward. He is so beautiful in his desire to be there for her and he longs to give her pleasure and be the lover of her dreams. When I guide him how to massage her slowly, connecting fully so it creates great arousal through anticipation, at first it feels to him like he is barely moving, barely doing anything, but to her, the slow moving connection of his hands on her body is sheer ecstasy.

I hear men say they want to learn to perform better. A woman does not want performance, she wants connection. The best Gift a man can give his woman is to learn the art of truly taking his time; to be fully present, to connect deeply, opening her more and more to surrender, slowly, skillfully, and artfully.

The Masculine is structure and holds space. The Feminine is flow and movement. If you look at a beach, the shore and the rocks would be the Masculine aspect, while the water is the Feminine.

If you look at a rose, the Masculine aspect would be the structure of the petals. The Feminine aspect would be the scent that flows from the rose.

Beautiful Masculine Lover, hold space for her. Penetrate her heart and soul, open her with just a gaze, by words spoken, a gentle touch, a slow caress. Take your time to the point where her body is aching for you. When the Feminine feels savored in this way, you open her to God and her surrender and her expression fills you with light.

Beautiful Feminine Lover, extend your invitation to him

through the sparkle in your eyes and the flow of your body language. Give him your trust. Surrender and open to him. Enthusiastically express your beautiful Divine Feminine erotic self with him, and together enter dimensions of Divine Union, devotion and extraordinary ecstasy.

The dance between the Masculine and Feminine is one of the most delicious, expansive experiences of being a human. We are a Gift to one another. Show up for one another fully with compassion, passion, and kindness, honoring the uniqueness and polarity of one another. Explore the possibilities within the dance. Merge your minds, hearts, bodies, and souls in ecstatic Divine Union.

THE FIVE ELEMENTS OF SEXUAL EXPRESSION™

I am mostly monogamous by nature. I say "mostly" because even when in a relationship, I still enjoy the freedom of expressing friendly affection toward other men in the form of a hug or a kiss. I jokingly call myself polyaffectionate. There was a brief time in 2014 when I explored polyamory. Translated polyamory means "multiple loves." Unlike swinging or being promiscuous, polyamory is when you have multiple sexual lovers at the same time and you have a genuine heart connection with each of them.

Through my polyamorous experience, I gained an awareness and wisdom that gave birth to what I call, *The Five Elements of Sexual Expression*™. This has become a wonderful tool I use with my clients to assist them in experiencing more depth and sexual fulfillment, physically, emotionally and spiritually.

My polyamorous experience involved three lovers. I was with the first man months before the other two and it was my connection with him that led to meeting them. He is a Shaman, Holy Man and a Healer.

We were only intimate a few times as our paths were focused in different directions. When we met I had not had a man penetrate me in five years due to the pain I would feel during intercourse caused by the common menopausal symptom, the thinning of the vaginal walls.

During our first time together, he spent hours throughout the night giving me energy healing and touch along my spinal column while I slept. In the morning after I woke, the touch turned to a more sensual stimulating arousal. He then gently massaged what he called a Sacred oil onto my yoni. Then we had intercourse and although he was well endowed, there was absolutely no pain, only pure pleasure. It was magical.

During our second time together, it was I who devoted more time to touching him. I intentionally channeled healing energy through my hands as I touched him sexually while surrendering to the love of the Divine moving through me while bringing him to orgasm. He shared that what he experienced was truly profound. Through my touch he felt layers of healing take place, clearing sexual wounding of multiple generations of ancestors before him.

For privacy and simplicity of communication, I will now call him my Healing Friend.

- **Healing** is one of *The Five Elements of Sexual Expression*™.

I REMAIN dear friends with my Healing Friend. A few months after we shared intimacy he introduced me to one of his friends visiting from out of town who needed a place to stay. My Healing Friend knew that I had space in my home, so he asked if his friend could stay with me for a few days. I agreed.

As thanks for opening my home to him, his friend offered to give me a massage. I accepted his offer. The massage was wonderful and evolved into sensuality, then sexual touch. His stay in my home became extended and for a short while, we continued to be sexual partners.

We spent time hanging out, sharing laughter and conversation. He had a very different energy from my Healing Friend. He was a little rougher around the edges. He only massaged me that one time. Our connection was one of friendship and mutual respect. With him, the sex was more raw and primal based. This is something I welcomed and craved due to so many years of not being able to be physically penetrated by a man.

From this point on, I will call him my Primal Friend.

- **Primal Expression** is one of *The Five Elements of Sexual Expression*™.

PRIMAL EXPRESSION
"Your Primal Expression is not separate from Spiritual Alignment.

It is an integral part of the tapestry of your Divine Creation.
Be playful with it. Dance to drums.
Get your hands in the soil. Roll in the mud.
Howl at the moon. Express it!"
~ Sacred Sexual Enlightenment Wisdom Cards

❦

WITHIN A COUPLE DAYS of my Primal Friend staying at my home, he invited a friend of his to come and visit. One night while the three of us were sitting around the living room talking, I shared that I had a stiff neck. This new friend offered to massage my neck, so I sat on the floor as he sat on the sofa. His hands felt wonderful as the stiffness in my neck melted away.

My Primal Friend observed the connection that his friend and I shared and suggested that we go into my room, so he could give me a more complete session on my massage table. We agreed.

This massage lasted for about two hours. His large hands were strong, intuitive and nurturing as he connected with my body. We became lovers that night.

For a time both this new lover and my Primal Friend stayed in my home at the same time. They were never lovers in my bed simultaneously, but for a few weeks, my time being sexual with them was interwoven between the two. Each knew that I was having sex with the other and all three of us were in full agreement of the connection we shared. I felt honored and indulged in this new polyamorous experience.

I remained lovers with this new friend for a few months.

I remained lovers with him the longest because of the quality of nurturing that I felt with him. We slept together so beautifully and peacefully as he held me through the night with his long limbs wrapped around my body. I loved being wrapped up in his warmth in this way. His tender heart and kindness were also nurturing.

He loved to give massages and gave them often. His nurturing was healing. He is my Nurturing Friend.

- **Nurturing** is one of *The Five Elements of Sexual Expression*™.

SHORTLY AFTER MY time of intimacy was complete with all three men and I reflected back on the experience. I realized how each man was more prominent in a different quality than the other two. Together all three provided a beautiful connection.

Each had an inner beauty and they were also beautiful on the outside. They each had brown skin in different tones and strong, lean muscular bodies. I called them my three Kings.

One Gifted me primarily with the expression of Healing; another with Primal Expression, and the other with Nurturing.

With all three, I felt connection. Without connection, intimacy never would have happened with any of them.

- **Connection** is one of *The Five Elements of Sexual Expression*™.

CONNECTION MUST ALWAYS BE present when expressing any of the other elements. Connection with your love. When you recognize you as the love of your life, you see and feel the love in everyone else. Your connection with them will always be beautiful, whether fleeting or long term. Without self-love you risk attracting distorted or unhealthy relationships as your reflection. It starts with your love within and then expands outward from there. Sacred Sexuality is the integration of your love and connection with self, the other and God Source into your sexual experience.

During the early stages of creating *The Five Elements of Sexual Expression*™, I merged healing and nurturing as one element, as they overlap. Nurturing is healing and healing is nurturing. That left me with three elements, but intuitively I knew there was another. I just wasn't sure what it was. So, I searched within and asked for the answer to come through me.

Of course, it was right there in front of me! I had forgotten to look at what element I brought to the equation that was more prominent than what my three lovers had.

Playfulness was my Gift to them. Playfulness is a prominent expression of mine in all aspects of my life. Relationships can be intense at times and serious issues will come up. Sex can take you to some deep places. Just remember to not take things too seriously all the time. Life is supposed to be fun. Sex is supposed to be fun. Be Playful with it.

- ***Playfulness*** is one of *The Five Elements of Sexual Expression*™.

OVER TIME, I split healing and nurturing as individual elements. I do this to encourage you to explore intentionally activating and channeling your sexual energy as a source of healing as I experienced with my Healing Friend. I invite you to sometimes integrate this into your sexual expression, like a meditation practice.

Here is a healing practice you can try: Before touching your partner, take a moment to breathe deep relaxing breaths and visualize Divine love light moving through you. First feel this light enter your heart, then out through your hands. Integrate your breath to help you move your energy in this way. Touch your partner from a space of pure giving as they surrender to receive without reciprocation. Do not see them as in need of healing, rather see them as whole, no matter what.

Touch them sensuously and sexually from this space, as they breathe in and receive your healing loving touch. Take turns with this, with one as the giver and the other completely receiving. Guide them to take deep breaths to receive the energy more fully. If you are an energy healer, this practice will come especially easy for you. Sexual energy is potent. Whatever intention we infuse it with, it amplifies it. Activating sexual energy for healing from a space of love is a powerful practice.

"Wherever you are, and whatever you do, be in love."
~ Rumi

THE FIVE ELEMENTS of Sexual Expression™ are:

- Healing
- Nurturing
- Primal Expression
- Connection
- Playfulness

During the birthing of *The Five Elements of Sexual Expression*™, I experienced them with three lovers, as was my journey. However, you can easily experience all Five Elements to equal degrees with one lover. It will be a dance between the five, with some elements being more prominently expressed than the others at different times.

Try this exercise: write the Five Elements down on a piece of paper and next to each one, write how expressed you are on a scale of 1 to 10. This gives you a clear visual of where you need to give more attention and expression.

If you're not on the same page with what you want to express in the heat of the moment, it creates disconnect. For example, if one partner wants to be more primal in their expression and initiates sex from this space while at the same time the other partner is longing for healing and nurturing, they may pull away. Here it is best to fulfill the desire for healing and nurturing first. Then from there, they will be more open to shift into primal expression. Be aware and communicate.

You don't have to do a meditative style healing practice every time as I described above for the other to feel your healing energy. Remember nurturing is naturally healing, so simply by giving focus on nurturing, they will feel the energy of healing in your embrace and in your giving.

If you resist the expression of one of the Five Elements, embrace this as an opportunity to look within and discover why you are holding back. It's likely you are holding back out of protection. As you discover and acknowledge the root source of what you are protecting, you'll likely find an unresolved wound there. It is not our nature to hold back on any of *The Five Elements of Sexual Expression*™. When we do, we are suppressing an aspect of ourselves.

When all Five of these Elements are expressed, sex is so beautiful and fulfilling on every level.

SUMMARY

Beloved, cherish and savor your sexual expression as the precious Gift of love that it is, in all its dimensions. As you do this, you will experience a deeper love of self, with Source, and with your partner(s).

You get to envision and create what you desire in this dream called life, that includes creating and living a joyful, blissful love life, beyond your imagination, spiritually, sexually and emotionally, with or without a partner.

APPLYING THE 1ST SACRED LAW TO THE WORKPLACE

Truths of past abuse are being exposed as women have become unmuted. Through the rise of the Me Too and Time's Up Movement, business leaders and film producers fear the possibility of sexual harassment suits and want to ensure a harmonious work environment between men and women.

Applying the Gift to the workplace is simple. Recognize the unique gifts that the Masculine and Feminine bring to the table. The Masculine loves competition and they have the Gift of focus. The workplace is a space where they get to play out their hunt and kill instinct. The Feminine thrives through collaboration, versus competition. Compassion and intuition are qualities of the Divine Feminine. Providing safety is a quality of the Divine Masculine.

Merge the Gifts and qualities of both the Masculine and Feminine/men and women. Work together respecting one another with kind, compassionate, mindful communication. When you ensure a safe, harmonious work environment, it also contributes to productivity and prosperity.

Women who have been wounded by abuse do not need to be consoled with good intentioned attempts to understand. They need good men to stand by their side insisting on dignity, honor and protection.

These Four Sacred Laws are primarily written for lovers; however, the same principles apply to all relationships. The Masculine dominated way of running the world no longer works. A Feminine dominated world is not the answer either. Women and men must stand side by side, honoring one another and celebrating the unique Gifts we have to offer.

The Masculine and Feminine cannot be split or separated. We have both within us. We are a reflection of one another and what a beautiful combination we are! Coming together in union is the only way we can thrive, whether it is in romantic relationships, in the workplace or as a society in general.

CHAPTER 6

Forgiveness

The 2nd Sacred Law of Sexual Enlightenment is **FORGIVENESS**

FORGIVENESS
"Self-love, Spiritual alignment and Peace
within the very energy that creates us
are necessary nourishment to thrive
and savor a more joyful existence.
Forgiveness of others and self may be
the Gift you need to take you there."
~ Sacred Sexual Enlightenment Wisdom Cards

THE GIFT OF FORGIVENESS

Forgiveness is a gift you give yourself. You must be at peace with the past and everyone in it, to be fully at peace and happy in the present. Whether your past wounds are as recent as yesterday or as distant as childhood, if you are holding onto any form of resentment, hurt or anger, you are holding yourself captive inside the experience that originally wounded you. That part of you will remain stuck within the energy of this experience until you release it, let it go and clear it at the source.

"Forgiveness is the moment we stop wishing the past was different". ~ Don Miguel Ruiz Jr; Circle of Fire - 2018

When we hold onto pain and emotional residue from the past, it maintains an unhealthy energetic connection with the other person or persons who were involved in that experience with us.

This is a journey I know well, as I had my own emotional wounding to clear and free myself from. It is why I am so passionate about helping others do the same and why I became a facilitator of emotional healing through breath work and other methods. I found what works and I love to share it.

If you feel resistance in fully expressing your sexually, it is likely from lack of emotional peace and contraction in your sexual body, due to a layer of Forgiveness that has yet to take place. Do you still carry emotional wounding from past abuse or trauma? Are you ready to let it go? If you no longer want to feel the same thing that happened to you, then forgive.

"HEALING
Heal your Heart.
Transform painful experience into wisdom.

*Be in Sexual Expression that is Healing
and nourish your soul with its beauty."*
~ *Sacred Sexual Enlightenment Wisdom Cards*

If you struggle with Forgiveness whether it is sexually related or not, in this chapter I will share with you a simple process that will help you quickly shift your perspective so you can move through the Forgiveness process with greater ease. Once you reach the point where you are no longer emotionally triggered and no longer feel pain, what you are left with is pure wisdom.

This is the beauty of Forgiveness—your pain transcends into wisdom. When this happens, it liberates you. You are no longer holding back to protect this vulnerable aspect of yourself, You become free to create the masterpiece out of your life that your heart yearns for.

Something as simple as getting cut off in traffic or having an experience with a cranky sales clerk, can cause a disruption in the way you feel if you allow it to. The ability to forgive in the moment with day-to-day experiences is a more peaceful way of living versus getting caught up in reactivity.

Every breath of your life is too precious to allow it to be contaminated by bitterness, resentment or sadness. These emotions are not to be judged, but you don't want to stay in the toxicity of them either. They can teach you much about yourself as you move through them and come out the other side.

Anger and grief are natural human emotions that must be expressed and released. Express it, don't repress it. Repression leads to depression. Over time, if you don't take steps to free yourself from the emotional charge of a past event, you reach a point when you are no longer a victim and you are playing a victim.

Releasing anger in a healthy way that does not hurt yourself or another is transformational. Moving through your grief and sadness, allowing the tears to flow, is very healing. What you want to be cautious of is getting caught up in the healing journey so much that you are consistently in a state of healing, recycling the same pain. With skilled professional help, you can move through the pain, release it and claim a life rich with deeper love, pleasure and peacefulness.

When I facilitate my healing work, the last thing I want is for my clients to become dependent on me. All the methods I use are swift, effective and powerful and some can be taught as a method of self-healing without the dependency of a facilitator.

FORGIVENESS FOR HEALTH

In chapter *1*, I shared how the grackle came when I called out to God for help. I shared how the teaching of the grackle is to release emotional congestion of the past before it manifests into physical illness, so you can move forward into the future. Forgiveness not only contributes to emotional health, it contributes to physical health.

Dr. Masaru Emoto revealed scientific evidence in his book, *The Hidden Messages in Water* that proved our thoughts and feelings directly affect the molecular structure of water.

He wrote words of hate on pieces of paper and attached them to jars of water. He then photographed these water molecules and revealed that they had turned into dark, distorted formations in response to the negativity projected toward it. He also wrote words of love and attached them to the water. When he photographed these molecules, they were beautiful crystalline formations resembling snowflakes.

Because 70 percent of your physical body is water, your body responds to your thoughts and feelings the same as the water in Dr. Emoto's experiment. When you hold onto bitterness, you literally distort the molecular structure of your body. Lack of Forgiveness festers and creates a dis-ease in your vibrational field, directly affecting your physical body. Dis-ease leads to disease. Forgiveness literally prevents disease.

Love your body as if it were an innocent child. Your body is never to blame. It is innocent. If you have more fat on your body than you'd like, it's not your body's fault. Observe if you say things like, "I hate my thighs" or "I hate my belly." It is unkind to say such things to your body. There is beauty in every body shape and size. Stop comparing. Observe your body's beauty and love your body for the shape it is with all of its imperfections.

Your body is so loyal. It works so hard to take care of you, even when you abuse it. Your body is a miracle of creation, constantly renewing itself by creating new cells every day and processing what you feed it. Forgive yourself if you have been hard on your body and begin a new relationship with your precious body temple. This will open you to a deeper sense of self-love, which in turn will contribute to your emotional and physical health.

ECSTATIC SELF-LOVE

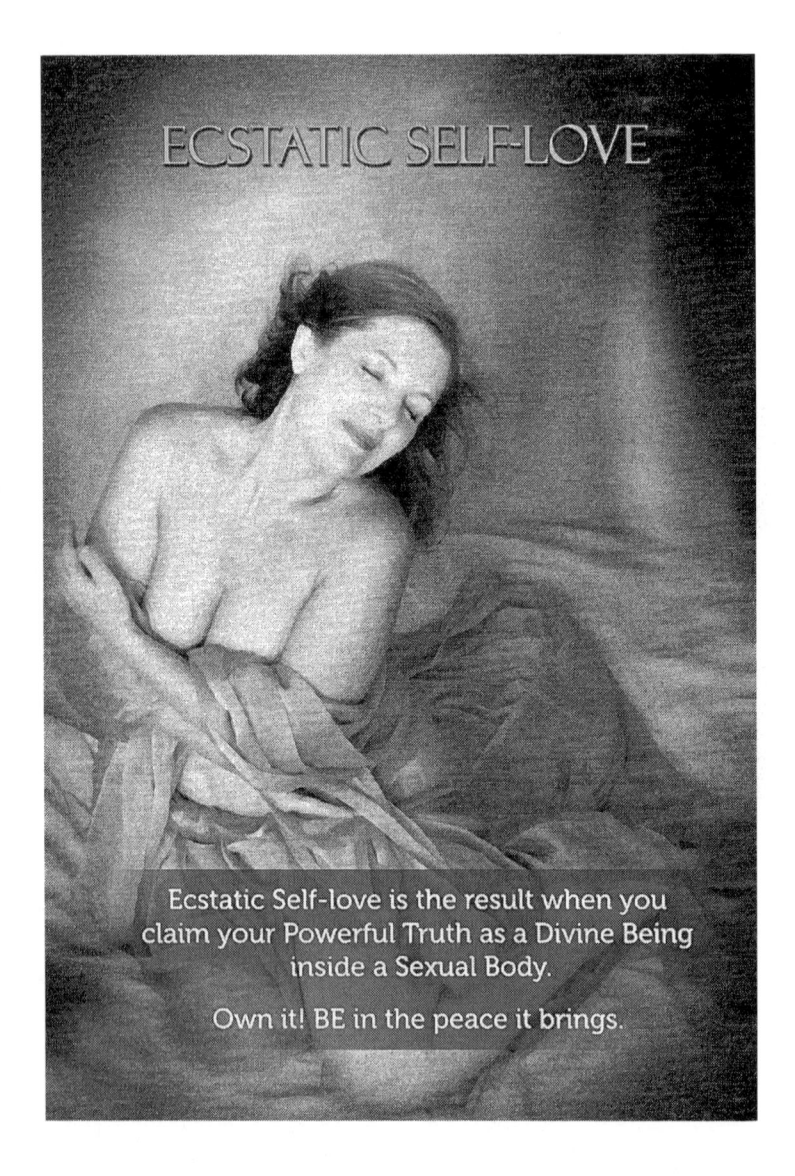

Ecstatic Self-love is the result when you claim your Powerful Truth as a Divine Being inside a Sexual Body.

Own it! BE in the peace it brings.

Your body is designed for pleasure. Give more pleasure to yourself, whether through dance, sports, being in nature, being in water, or sharing your body with someone who will honor, love and appreciate you and your body exactly as you are.

Giving pleasure to your body is an act of self-love. Self-love is easy when you acknowledge the truth of who you are as a Divine being, inside a physical sexual body. It also makes the Forgiveness process much easier.

Through self-love, you are never lonely because so many are drawn to your light. From this space you're already full of love, so you don't choose to be with another because you feel you need it. You choose them because they reflect your love and because it gives you joy to be in their presence and to bear witness to one another's life.

MARRIAGE & OTHER INTIMATE RELATIONSHIPS

Forgiveness of a past relationship with a spouse, boyfriend or girlfriend that resulted in wounding or bitterness is crucial to being able to fully show up in a new relationship. Holding onto emotional garbage of the past contaminates relationships in the present. Forgiveness makes space for peacefulness and is a gift of love to you and for them.

Do you still blame an ex for your unhappiness? Do you talk about what a lousy lover they were? Ask yourself, if this is the frequency you want to be dialed into? For example, if you want to receive music that plays on 99.9 FM radio, you cannot set the dial to 105 AM and expect to receive your music. The frequencies do not match up. The same is true for love.

It can be easy to believe if you are with the right partner, you can be happy, but if you still complain about your ex-relationship, and hook up with a new one, it won't be long before you're complaining about them as well. You cannot open to love when you are resentful. Love expands, resentment contracts. Which one do you want to dial into?

"No one can make me feel inferior without my consent."
~ Eleanor Roosevelt

If you feel inferior due to the words or actions of an ex, you're making an agreement to feel this way. I recently attended the Circle of Fire Gathering hosted by Don Miguel Ruiz and his sons. Don Miguel Ruiz Jr asked us, do we give permission to ourselves to write our own story? Are we willing to remove what is not contributing to our story? Are we willing to surrender our poison and surrender our doubt? I love how simple and powerful these questions are. Our life is a dream that we create for ourselves, and this dream is our art. What is the vision you dream for yourself? How is your art unfolding? If there is something in your dream you do not like, remove it. Create your art with love.

If your relationship with your ex is unpleasant but they're still in your life because you parent children together, you get to choose whether or not you react to their opinions of you. What they say and do is a projection of their reality, not yours. Be immune to them.

At the core of all unpleasant behavior is a wound, so forgive. Teach your children how to be happy by choosing happiness for you. Gift you and your children with this. Hopefully your ex will follow your example and give them the same gift. Just don't have expectations. Focus on you and your dream. You can't control theirs.

Your past is just the way it is. Accept it. Learn from it. It doesn't exist anymore. Bless those who contributed to it. It has served you on your journey of acquiring new wisdom. Forgive and focus on what's good in the present.

If you want to attract a new loving, healthy, sexually vibrant relationship, then give that to yourself first. Be loving, adoring, kind and giving to your greatest love of all… you! Create a vibrant loving sexual relationship with you! Emanate in that frequency with you and you will attract it in another. Two people emanating in this space are the ideal foundation for sharing the ultimate love life together.

FAMILY LEGACY

What is the legacy you inherited around your sexual story? Belief systems are often ingrained from our parents and/or religious teachings. Are you holding onto a belief that is not serving you, interfering with your ability to experience a vibrant, happy sacred sex life with another?

A belief can only exist as long as you give it a "yes." It is an illusion that you can shatter if you choose. Why not believe what brings you joy? When you feel joy, you are in your truth. Joy is when your human self is in alignment with your Divine self. That's why it feels so good.

"In the Dream of the Planet, we have the need to justify everything — to make everything good or bad or right or wrong, when it is just the way it is, period. Humans accumulate a lot of knowledge; we learn all those beliefs, morals and rules from our family, society, religion. And we base most of our behavior, most of our feelings on that knowledge. We create angels and demons, and of course, sex becomes the biggest demon in hell. Sex is the biggest sin of the humans, when the human body is made for sex.

You are a biological, sexual being, and that is just the way it is. Your body is so wise. All that intelligence is in the genes, in the DNA. The DNA doesn't need to understand or justify everything; it just knows. The problem is not with sex. The problem is the way we manipulate the knowledge and our judgments, when there is really nothing to justify. It's so hard for the mind to surrender, to accept that it's just the way it is. We have a whole set of beliefs about what sex should be, about how relationships should be, and these beliefs are completely distorted."

~ Don Miguel Ruiz; from *The Mastery of Love*

EVEN IF YOUR parents did their best to provide a loving home for you, Forgiveness of parents may still be something you want to explore. This is not about making anyone wrong or passing blame. We're all figuring it out as we go, and a well-intentioned parent does the best they can with what they know. Understanding the good intentions behind the limiting belief you inherited gives clarity to the situation and sheds light on how to move through it and rise above it.

Two of the first questions I ask my clients who come for sexual healing or to learn about Tantric Sexuality is, "What was your relationship like with your parents?" and "What was your parents' relationship like with one another?" These two questions tell me so much about the individual, and they give me strong clues that help me to know the best way for me to proceed with the session.

In the first five years of offering private bodywork sessions, my clients were primarily men. I offered massage integrated with energy healing and Tantric Sexuality teachings. I would guide them to harness their sexual energy by opening their heart center, interweaving it with their breath, and feelings of self-love. One of the most powerful healing sessions was with a physically very large man who came to see me wanting to learn about Tantric Sexuality. Let's call this man Ryan.

After I asked the initial questions about his relationship with his parents, I discovered that Ryan had suffered severe verbal abuse by his father when he was a boy. It was obvious there was still deep wounding there. With this knowledge, I knew the session needed to go in a different direction than a basic lesson in breath work and the channeling of sexual energy. I took him through the Forgiveness process I am sharing with you later in this chapter, and a deep healing process that involves rewriting the parent story.

The nervous system doesn't know if an experience is real or make-believe. It responds the same, regardless. This is also why it's so important for actors to learn how to clear and neutralize their energy after acting a traumatic scene, so the energy of the make-believe trauma does not integrate into the cells of their body. During my session with Ryan, I guided him through a process where we created a healthy new father story while I stimulated his spinal column through touch. His nervous system recognized this story as real, allowing the unhealthy father memory to fade as we integrated a new loving father story.

As we moved through this process, I held Ryan in my arms as his large body shook with emotion, with tears flowing down his face as his father wounds healed. He shared that during our session, it was the closest he had ever felt to his father.

Ryan came back for two more sessions. By the third session, he was finally ready to learn how to integrate his breath and his sexual energy. I waited until he was in a new space of peacefulness in his emotional body, more confident and self-loving. From this space, he was able to show up and work with his own energy free from feelings of self-judgment, and free from the sound of a judgmental father's voice playing out in his head. From this space, he embodied and activated his sexual energy, so it was Spiritually aligned, whole and joyful.

Ryan's life was forever changed. He was so grateful that I took the sessions in a different direction than he expected. Forgiving his father and forgiving himself was transformational and opened him to a beautiful new realm of possibility for future relationships.

Abuse by anyone, especially a parent whether it is verbal or physical can create wounding that stays with a person well into adulthood until they have the proper guidance or inner breakthrough to free them from the pain of the experience. Forgiveness is always a key element to this healing process.

Even with loving, well-intentioned parents, the relationship that Mom and Dad had with one another may not have been ideal. As children, our most powerful learning is by example. If you grew up in a home with parents who were not affectionate with one another, this may have created a subconscious belief this is what intimacy is.

Clearing a constricting belief inherited from family around sexuality follows the same process as clearing a belief inherited from conservative religious teachings. The religion you grew up with, was present in your home and integrated into your family life.

I developed a simple one-hour process called *Heal Your Sexual Legacy*™ that I facilitate privately or in groups. It is just as effective done in person as it is through video. Part of this process involves writing a Forgiveness letter. I also have a Home Study version of this process in video format available on my website, which you can access at: Jaitara.com/Store

SEXUAL ABUSE

Sexual abuse is an act of violence. Any unwanted sexual contact is categorized as sexual violence, this includes unwanted fondling, kissing, rubbing or any other sexual act. Stalking or distributing intimate video recordings is sexual violence, even if there is no physical contact. All of these examples are serious offenses and can be very damaging to the victim.

With so many rapes going unreported, the percentages I am giving you about female and male rape are approximate. Based on the findings of the National Center for Victims of Crime, one out of five women and one out of twenty men have endured childhood sexual abuse. The percentages of sexual abuse continue to increase for both men and women into college age and beyond. Are you one of these men or women? Does your past abuse experience still haunt you?

Almost every woman has experienced some form of sexual harassment. Forgiveness is a powerful step toward healing sexual harassment and abuse. It can also be very challenging, especially if the abused was a child at the time.

In addition to breath work, when I work with clients who have experienced trauma such as rape and abuse, I also integrate a powerful revolutionary verbal guided process that is profound in its swiftness and effectiveness for permanently dissolving inner conflict and the emotional triggers around their trauma. In as little as fifteen minutes it can dissolve the emotional trigger attached to the trauma.

I know fifteen minutes seems unrealistic, I didn't believe it myself when I first heard of this process, but it's true. For some, it may take up to forty-five minutes, which is still a short while for such a dramatic shift. This method is effective both in person and through online live video facilitation.

If you still carry a charge around a rape or abusive incident and you wish to receive one of these sessions, go to: Jaitara.com/Connect to arrange for an appointment.

Much love.

STILLNESS
"Be in Stillness.
Start your day connecting
and listening to the breath.
Meditate, chant mantras.
Appreciate all the good in your life
and the blessing of your body."
~ Sacred Sexual Enlightenment Wisdom Cards

I'm able to share my story of sexual exploitation from my adolescence so openly because I freed myself from the emotional residue and the emotional triggers of that experience. Forgiveness did not erase the memory of my experience. It set me free from the emotional reactivity to it. What I am left with is pure wisdom and lightness, and the knowledge that makes it possible for me to write this book and help others through their healing journey.

Sexual energy is at the root of your very existence. You must have healthy roots to fully thrive. If you feel you can't forgive someone because you don't feel they deserve Forgiveness, then forgive them as a gift to yourself. Give yourself this gift of inner peacefulness. Transcend your pain to wisdom, lightness and love.

ROOTS

*"Sexual Energy is the Root of your Creative Force.
Just like a tree, your roots must be nourished, vibrant
and healthy to reveal all you're here to Express and BE.
Take care and feed your Roots through
Healing, Nurturing and Connection."*
~ Sacred Sexual Enlightenment Wisdom Cards

FORGIVENESS OF SELF

One of the most confusing aspects of sexual abuse is that often pleasure was involved in the experience. The nerve endings that create physical pleasure still work the same whether it is abusive or consensual. This is where the challenge of Forgiving self often comes into play in relation to an abusive experience.

I remember when Oprah first went public with her experience of childhood sexual abuse in 1999, sharing how she was raped at age nine, then again up until age fourteen. She expressed that much of her confusion was because she was being touched in a way that physical pleasure was stimulated. So, she blamed herself for years, even though she was a child at the time of the abuse.

Oprah's sharing was powerful. It freed many from the guilt they too carried from an abuse experience. I was one of them. Although I didn't feel it immediately, it created a shift and an opening in my energy. Two weeks later I had my *Day of the Grackle* experience.

When I was manipulated into teenage prostitution, even

though deep down in my soul I was screaming "NO," I was still experiencing physical pleasure. For twenty-seven years I secretly carried shame and self-judgment and a belief that I had lower morals than most people. I was afraid to share my secret, even with my closest of friends. My distorted belief was that if they knew about my past, they wouldn't want to be my friend. It was such a gift when I saw the billboard that day in the subway station. It was like the Universe had magically orchestrated my awakening.

By the year 1999, I was at an age when my friends had sixteen-year-old daughters. Through my connection with them, I woke up to the reality of how young I had actually been when my abuse took place. When we are young, whether a small child or a teenager, in our mind we feel older than we really are.

So many child abuse victims hold themselves responsible and in a space of self-blame well into adulthood. A part of us stays stuck in the mindset when the abuse took place. A part of us also stays stuck in the time before it took place when it still felt safe. We remain there until we can set ourselves free from the pain of the experience. Forgiveness of self is one of the most powerful steps to being liberated from the trauma of sexual abuse.

BREATHE
"Does sexual wounding or shadows of the past mask or inhibit your expression in the present? Learn to Breathe the Cleansing Breath for healing and emotional liberation, so you can savor the fruit of life and we experience the full truth and juiciness of you."
~ Sacred Sexual Enlightenment Wisdom Cards

I became a facilitator of breath work because it's what worked for me. Through the breath, I forgave everyone from my past and myself. I released all the blame and emotional garbage that had to be cleared out of my system, so I can live fully at peace in the now. Breath work literally saved my life. It cleared the emotional residue from my body on a cellular level, permanently releasing the past pain, and replacing it with love, lightness, aliveness and wisdom. That is the power of breath.

ENERGY IN MOTION

E-motion is "energy in motion." Breath is a brilliant tool and vehicle for moving energy through our body. The breath can be used to channel sexual energy for the purpose of increasing pleasure and spiritual connection. I share this in great detail in the chapter on the *4th Sacred Law, The Invitation.*

The breath is like a built in vacuum cleaner for healing and clearing suppressed or built up emotional energy. Yet, few have learned how to activate and utilize its full power. I adore the breath. It is always a great honor for me to facilitate the breath and witness my clients go through the transformational shift breath work sessions provide.

In almost every session I facilitate, I hear my clients say, "I didn't even know that was in there." The most powerful experience they often have, is the clearing of energy they did not know was inside them. When something is emotionally painful, it can be blocked out and forgotten. It's the soul's way of protecting itself. The body and soul have great wisdom. During an emotional healing breath work session, only what we are ready to handle at that moment, is what

will come to the surface and be released. That is the wisdom of the body and soul.

A great way to move through the Forgiveness process on your own is to shift your perspective. Often, the abused still perceives their past abuser as someone who is overpowering, even though many years may have passed since the experience. I'm sharing a simple process that will help you or someone you know shift your perspective to make Forgiveness easier to move through.

Read the following process, then close your eyes and take yourself through it. If you prefer to have my voice guide you, then go to Jaitara.com/Store to access a free audio on my website where my voice will guide you through the process.

FORGIVENESS PROCESS

- Begin by closing your eyes. Take deep relaxing breaths in through your nose and out through your mouth. Connect only with the sound of your breath going in and out of your body, fully tuning into this connection.
- Once you feel this connection, hold a vision of the past abuser in your mind. See them as a frozen snapshot versus a moving video. By seeing

just a still image of their face, you are not reenacting the experience. See their face as they look in the current day. If you don't know what they look like now, then imagine it.
- Now imagine what they looked like five years prior to this. Once you clearly see this image, then imagine what they looked like ten years prior to that. Again, see this as a still snapshot image.
- Keep taking them back in time until you can visualize and imagine what they looked like as a teenager.
- Now take them back in time even more until you see them as a ten-year-old child.
- Now imagine them as a five-year-old child and ask yourself, "What was their environment like? How were they being loved? What were they being taught?" As you visualize this image and feel into this, you probably can see this five-year-old child was not being loved in the way a five-year-old child should be loved and deserves to be loved.
- It's likely they were not in a healthy environment and not being taught what a five-year-old child must be taught to have a healthy and happy perspective on life. An individual who is emotionally whole, raised in a conscious loving home does not grow up to be someone who intentionally inflicts pain onto another.
- So now as you've seen them as this five-year-old child, and you can imagine their environment,

now see them growing up and as a ten-year-old child with that same environment and experience, and then ask yourself, "What was their environment like? How were they being loved? What were they being taught?"
- Now see them as a teen and ask the questions again, "What was their environment like? How were they being loved? What were they being taught?"
- Now envision them growing into an adult whose childhood wounding was left unresolved. Now you have a much different perspective as you view this person.

THIS DOES NOT CONDONE what they did. As adults we must take responsibility for our actions and for healing our own wounds. What taking yourself through this process does is quickly shift your perspective of the abuser into one of greater compassion. Instead of seeing your abuser as someone with an overbearing power over you, you can now see them as a wounded five-year-old child.

Forgiveness does not justify what the abuser did, but this process will shift you from pointing a finger at *what*, to focusing on the *why*. At the root of the *why* is always a child with an unresolved wound. This is so simple and so effective in helping you move through Forgiveness. This shift in perspective is a powerful way to release bitterness and resentment you carry toward anyone from the past.

Remember, this Forgiveness process is intended for an experience that is past history. If you are currently still in an abusive situation, this process may help you feel a level of compassion for the abuser, but your priority must be focused on getting out of your situation. Seek the professional help you need to get away from your abuser and be safe.

Often bitterness and resentment are rooted in a desire to make them pay, to make it right, to make them suffer, to right the wrong. Yes, when someone commits a crime, it's important they be held responsible, however, carrying bitterness and resentment over the years will only hurt you the most. It will only hold you in a place of unhappiness and dis-ease that can eventually result in disease.

When you don't Forgive, you cut yourself off from the pleasure you can experience in this beautiful dream of life. When you cut yourself off from pleasure, you also teach by example. This pattern is not a healthy example for the generations who follow. So, Forgiveness is not only a gift you give to yourself, it is a gift you give to your children. As you come to peace with your past, then that peace becomes a vibration in their existence as well.

If Forgiveness has been a challenge for you, ask yourself, "Am I ready to let this go? Am I ready to give myself this freedom now? Am I ready to give myself this peace now?"

Take yourself through the Forgiveness process I just shared with you, right now. If you go to my website, you can access the free audio of my voice guiding you through it. It's time to set yourself free of the hold that they have on you.

If this doesn't apply to you, then I'm sure you know someone who can use help with this. This process is quick, easy and effective. Share it with them.

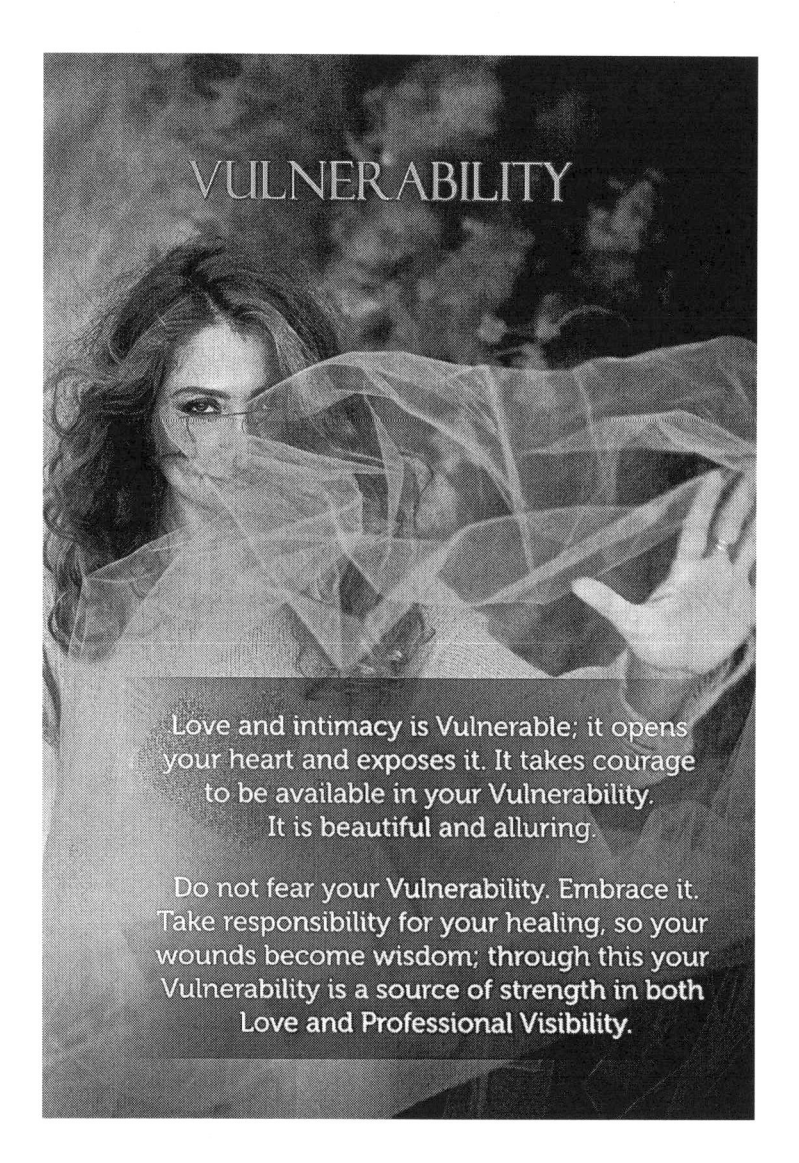

VULNERABILITY

Love and intimacy is Vulnerable; it opens your heart and exposes it. It takes courage to be available in your Vulnerability. It is beautiful and alluring.

Do not fear your Vulnerability. Embrace it. Take responsibility for your healing, so your wounds become wisdom; through this your Vulnerability is a source of strength in both Love and Professional Visibility.

Energy cannot be created and cannot be destroyed, but it can be transmuted. Look back and reflect upon all past relationships. As you take inventory, ask yourself if you feel any triggers or contraction in your body when you think of these people. If you do, there's still a layer of Forgiveness that needs to take place. With every layer of Forgiveness, I promise you it will be replaced with a new layer of inner peace, love, and lightness.

You came into this world as a beautiful innocent baby, who wanted to love, be loved, express love and experience joy. This reality is still true. Love and joy is your most natural state. Relationships are vulnerable. Love is vulnerable. When you love yourself first, you feel strong in your vulnerability, not fearful.

The experiences and the people you were exposed to as a child and the choices they made for you molded and shifted your reality, resulting in who you are now. You knew when you came into this body, this human experience had contrast and that you would make mistakes and experience emotional pain. Knowing all this, you still came here willingly, because you also knew how orgasmic life can be, starting with the body you inhabit.

Everything in creation on this beautiful planet is sensual and sexual. The more we can Forgive, the more alive we feel and can fully witness and experience the beauty of that. Be kind and loving with yourself.

I frequently receive comments on my peacefulness. I know the primary reason for this is because of the healing that has taken place at the core of my sexual life force energy. Forgiving those from my past and forgiving myself was a huge part of my healing journey, my liberation and a contribution to my peaceful state of being.

I love the beauty and healing powers of Mother Earth; being surrounded by trees, the peace of the forest, a beach, or a mountaintop. We are part of the Earth. Always maintain a connection with her. In this modern world of technology, it's so important that we do all we can to maintain this connection. She is called "Mother" for a reason. She feeds us, shelters us and gives us all we need to survive. She is nourishing, healing and nurturing. She is a part of us and so very beautiful. Open yourself to her. Connect with her. Be kind to her.

EARTH

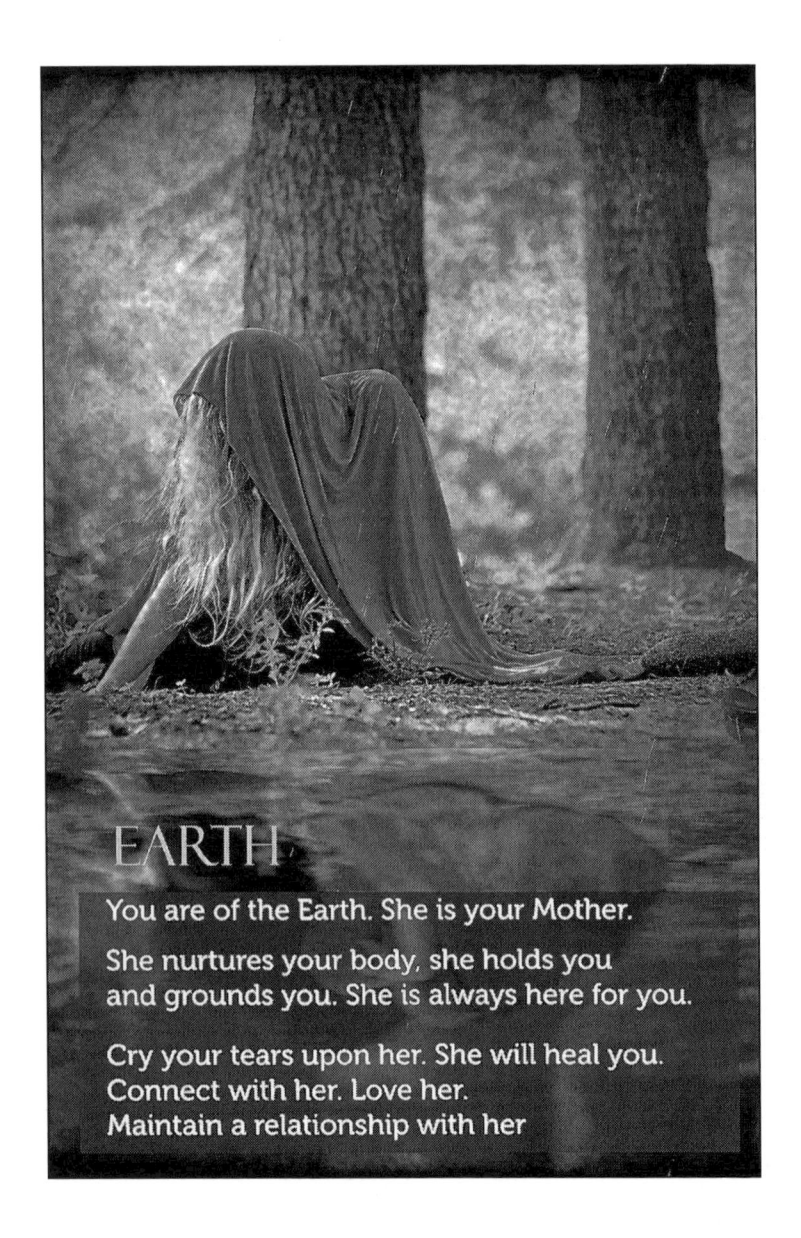

You are of the Earth. She is your Mother.

She nurtures your body, she holds you and grounds you. She is always here for you.

Cry your tears upon her. She will heal you.
Connect with her. Love her.
Maintain a relationship with her

SUMMARY

You have love, life and light within you, because love, life and light is what you are, and joy is your most natural state. That is your truth. If you don't feel it, giving yourself the gift of Forgiveness is a beautiful next step for you. Just because you exist, you are worthy and deserving off all the beauty, love, pleasure, goodness, and abundance that life has to offer.

Gift yourself with Forgiveness. Claim the peace, joy, aliveness, and wholeness that belong to you. What you experience and feel right now, directly influences what you experience tomorrow.

My love is with you. Blessings to you, Beloved One.

APPLYING THE 2ND SACRED LAW TO THE WORKPLACE

The larger the team in the workplace, the more diversity with regard to people's backgrounds, beliefs, personalities, and morals. It is natural for disputes and differences of opinions to arise. What is unacceptable is a display of disrespect toward one another.

When a dispute happens between colleagues, it creates disharmony between them as well as a tension in the air that affects everyone in the workplace. The sooner it is cleared, the better it is for your staff and for the company.

When I facilitate conflict resolution for couples, it is

never about blame or making one right or wrong. It is to ensure that what is being said is what is actually being heard and for both parties to take the time to really listen and respect the other's point of view. Then they come to mutual agreements that work for both parties. An exception is when one intentionally harms another. Here the couple is better off separating. The same is true for the workplace. If one is intentionally causing harm or sexually harassing, obviously that is reason for dismissal. If it is a dispute due to a different point of view, then work to establish harmony.

I recommend a "come clean" conversation between the parties involved or bring in a conflict resolution professional to help. Make sure that peaceful agreements are established, that also includes Forgiveness between the parties involved. Address it, forgive it and grow from it. Apply the lessons learned to reestablish a harmonious work environment.

CHAPTER 7

Responsibility

The 3rd Sacred Law of Sexual Enlightenment is
RESPONSIBILITY

SEXUAL ENLIGHTENMENT
"Sexual Enlightenment is the embodiment of our Divine Design
as an Awakened Sacred Being in a Sexual Body Temple.
Explore the beauty, sensuality, wisdom
and elegance of this with playful wonder.
Be in the expansiveness of this truth
and a luminous example for our youth."
~ Sacred Sexual Enlightenment Wisdom Cards

THIS SACRED LAW has many layers. The categories below are not in any particular order of importance. Each is unique and relevant.

RESPONSIBILITY TO TRUTH

We are Divine Beings and Sexual Beings. We have a Responsibility to honor this truth. In doing so we absolve the taboo around sexuality. Honoring this truth is not dependent upon the depth or length of a relationship. This applies no matter how brief the sexual encounter.

When you interweave your body and energy with another, you owe it to them and yourself to see them as the Divine Being they are. To see them as any less reflects how you see yourself. You also cheat them and you of the full beauty that your sexual encounter can bring. By failing to see the Divine in the one you share your body with, you dishonor the Divine in yourself. By honoring the Divinity in them and in you, the sexual experience carries a much higher vibration than sex void of this acknowledgment.

You came into this world as pure love. You are still pure love. This love connects us, and this love is the essence of the God Source energy that exists within each of us. You know when you are in alignment because you feel peace, kindness and joy within and it is easy to see the love in another.

Honor this truth of your Divinity. Recognize this in yourself and in your sexual partner, whether are you are together for a one-night stand or for the rest of your life. Show up fully, completely and compassionately.

"Namaste — I see you. I see you as a beautiful Divine being whose eternal consciousness pervades your body and mind, and is the light of your true self, shining across to mine. I bow to that transcendent being that is the real you."

~ Jeffrey Armstrong; *Spiritual Teachings of the Avatar*

RESPONSIBILITY OF HEALING

As I shared in the previous chapter on *Forgiveness*, if you still carry emotional residue from the past, it is your Responsibility to get the help you need to heal yourself. Only you can do this. Only you can take the necessary action and until you do, you risk contaminating current and future relationships with the shadows of your past.

If you are self-healing and find yourself stuck or blocked, seeking professional help is a responsible action to take. It is a kindness to yourself and to whomever you share your intimacy with.

RESPONSIBILITY OF COMMUNICATION

Being Responsible in our communication with one another is crucial in any relationship, especially one that involves sexuality. The following six topic are aspects of ***Responsibility of Communication.***

1. OUR YOUTH:

Sexual wholeness is imperative to the emotional well-being of our youth. They need those of us who are teachers, mentors and role models to include all aspects when teaching them about their sexual body... the full anatomy of both female and male; the beauty of sex, the sacredness of it, the pleasure, the power of it, the Responsibility of it, how to consciously communicate, and how to honor one another's boundaries.

Teaching our youth the path of Sacred Sexuality is key to their well-being. It starts with those of us who are adults stepping up and being responsible for our own sexual well-being, communication and truth.

Whether you are a parent or not, this Responsibility belongs to all of us. Imagine our future leaders maturing with this wisdom.

Responsibility to the youth is the aspect of this Sacred Law I am personally most passionate about. It is the *Big Why* and driving force behind my desire to do the work I do around sexuality. We have a huge Responsibility to our youth in the way we educate them about sexuality and there is room for a lot of improvement.

Even in today's advanced world, sex education is limited in what it teaches. Generally, sex-ed classes are just a biology lesson and even that is incomplete and anatomically incorrect. North American schools and to the best of my knowledge most countries on the planet eliminate the clitoris from the sex-ed biology lesson and diagrams as if it is nonexistent. At the time of writing this book, France is the only country I'm aware of that actually teaches about the clitoris in sex-ed classes.

In a Huffington Post article titled *What You Didn't Learn in Sex Ed*, they write that the book, *Hole's Essentials of Anatomy and Physiology* describes the clitoris as "about 2 centimeters long." Such inaccuracy is downright irresponsible! The tip of the clitoris on the exterior of the body may average that length, but that's like saying the totality of an iceberg is the piece you see sticking out of the water. The clitoris is actually around 4 inches in length. After menopause, it even grows an additional 2.5 times larger than when the same woman is a teenager.

The clitoris is the only human body part created for the sole purpose of pleasure, yet pleasure for both male and female is left out of the teachings in sex-ed. The large majority of women need clitoral stimulation to experience orgasm. Why is this not being taught?

In North America, teaching abstinence is still the primary teaching for birth control. Many schools do not even teach about contraceptives, how to apply a condom, or about consent. This focus on abstinence education does not increase the age for when the youth have their first sexual contact. It actually results in more teenage pregnancies, STIs, and abortions. Teenagers with hormones will be sexually active; that's a fact. To pretend otherwise is to be in denial and irresponsible.

Do we really want to live in a society where young women continue to be unfamiliar with their own bodies and young men and women continue to be in the dark when it comes to knowing how to be a lover? Do we want to continue to use anatomically incorrect biology lessons and fear as the primary teaching method around sexuality? It's time we teach about sexuality with truthfulness, accuracy and for it to be all-encompassing. It's the Responsible and enlightened thing to do.

We live in a time when everyone has easy access to pornography, and boys and girls are turning to porn as a source of sex education. They want to know what to do. Boys see the women in porn movies looking like they are having a good time, so they believe what they see is what women want. If you are a teen boy or young adult reading this, trust me, the large majority of what you see in porn is not what women want or how they want to be spoken to during sex.

With North American sex education not teaching about pleasure or that the clitoris even exists, combined with porn making it more about the man's pleasure than the woman's, most of the resources available on sex education and what qualifies as good sex are incomplete and distorted.

In 2013, when I was in Los Angeles, I became friends with an ex-porn star. He used to be a big name in the porn industry. He shared with me, when in the business he only worked for 20% of the business, because the other 80% was abusive toward women. He educates college students as a public speaker, informing the college boys that if they continue to watch porn, they will end up alone and become addicted to porn. He has a video online that teaches how to properly give oral sex to a woman. In this video, he shares that what is shown on camera is solely for entertainment and not what works for a woman in real life.

Girls need wise women to guide them and teach them about their sexuality. They must have permission to explore their own bodies and how to self-pleasure in a way that is physically, emotionally and spiritually fulfilling. Then by the time they are ready to share themselves with a partner, they know what they want, how to ask for it, how to provide guidance and how to give.

Some children are still shamed for touching their own bodies. This mindset is damaging. When they touch themselves, making the connection between their body, heart and soul, it does not lead to addictive tendencies. When a teen or young adult explores their body from a conscious space with a strong sense of self-love, self-worth, healthy body image, and self-awareness, they can grow into being a good lover and have a better chance of experiencing a healthy joyful relationship with themselves and another.

Boys need healthy men to guide and teach them about their sexuality. They must be taught the importance of consent, how to honor and communicate with the feminine. It's important they understand her anatomy as well as their own. Boys need healthy masculine guidance, so they have a better chance to grow up and be the healthy masculine themselves.

Girls and boys need to be taught the whole truth and the full dimension of who we are as spiritual beings inside these beautiful orgasmic, sexual bodies. Whether you are a parent or not, that's irrelevant, the youth are the Responsibility of all of us. The youth need us as a society to step up and be more responsible in our sexual education communication.

Until such resources are more readily available, reach out to the community around you. If you are a parent and it makes your child cringe to speak about sex with you, then connect with someone in your community who can, a friend, sister, brother, aunt or uncle.

Motivating the Teen Spirit is an organization I am familiar with that supports teens and helps them with teen issues. Motivating the Teen Spirit was founded by Lisa Nichols with Tia Ross as the program director. Knowing Tia as I do, I know they do good work with teens in the realm of healing from depression and trauma and personal empowerment as a whole. They have prevented many teen suicides from happening.

If you are a parent and communication is a challenge with your teen, or you are concerned about the direction they are going in, I highly recommend you get in touch with Motivating the Teen Spirit. They do not specialize in sexual education, however if the teens bring up the topic of sex, the facilitators will consciously discuss it with them and provide wise guidance.

2. FIRST TIME SEX:

Your first time with a new partner should feel beautiful and something you remember with a smile and warmth, even if it's your only time together. Spontaneity can be very sexy but before diving in with a new partner, taking time to openly communicate can save you from hurt, messiness and regret.

Communicate what your desires are or whether or not you have expectations. Is one of you in it for a casual encounter, while the other has deeper aspirations? If so, do not say "yes." Have integrity with yourself and the other person.

Are you both entering into this levelheaded, or is one of you going through depression and just seeking comfort? Are you feeling especially vulnerable due to a life crisis, death in the family, conflict with a loved one or loneliness?

Sex can be beautiful medicine, but communicate if either of you are feeling particularly vulnerable. If you are with someone in a vulnerable state and you think sex will make them feel better, think again. Unless they are giving you strong eye contact and an enthusiastic "YES," it's not a real "yes." If you are feeling vulnerable and you believe sex will make you feel better, take a moment to tune into the wisdom of your body. Does your body feel sexually excited, or contracted? If you feel contracted, sex is a temporary fix you may regret later.

We all have vulnerabilities but when a person is exceptionally tender, just cuddling can be a much better option than sex. Vulnerability can hinder a person's ability to say "no." They are longing for comfort, and touch is very comforting, so they may take it in any form it comes.

I remember feeling especially vulnerable when going through a difficult time ten years ago. A friend came over to comfort me and we ended up having sex. It was our first and only time. When he initiated sex I didn't say no, I responded so he believed I wanted it too. Though I responded, I was not an eye contact "yes." Cuddling would have comforted me much more. I really just needed to be held without feeling obligated to reciprocate.

When someone is going through a vulnerable time even if they believe they want sex, or if they seem responsive to it, wait. Just hold them. Give them a big comforting bear hug. This may even evoke tears to be held in a way where they feel safe and protected enough to relax and let go. If you are holding a woman, do not move your hands around their body, stroking them, as they may feel obligated to respond by stroking you back. Just hold them. Be present for them.

Maybe your perception is distorted through the influence of alcohol or drugs. If one or both of you are drunk or high wait until you are no longer under the influence before you have sex. Once you are clearheaded then you can talk about whether you still want to go there. Once the buzz is gone, the desire may be gone as well. Also, when under the influence important topics of discussion can be forgotten, such as STIs.

3. STIs:

The importance of communicating to a new sexual partner you have an STI (Sexually Transmitted Infection) is obvious, yet a Responsibility that can often go unspoken due to the stigma of shame around it, especially with the herpes simplex virus. Many people with herpes do not always share with their sexual partner they have it, due to fear of rejection and their awareness that the risk is quite low when the symptoms are dormant.

A large majority of the population has the herpes simplex virus. We must eliminate the shame around this. Herpes simplex virus 1 is the one that likes to live on the mouth area, known as cold sores or fever blisters. Herpes simplex virus 2 is almost the same as a cold sore, only it likes to live on the genital area. However, they can also switch places.

Why is it when most people see a cold sore on someone's lip, they don't give it much thought? Yet, if they discover they have a blister on their genitals, there is so much fear and shame around it? Herpes simplex type 1 can be transferred to the genitals through oral sex. The blister is the same. It's just on a different body part. Yet, it is uncommon for simplex 2 to transfer from the genitals to the mouth.

Those who do not have herpes, or believe that they don't, have a responsibility to educate themselves as much as those with it, if not more so. Lack of education can cause overreaction and unnecessary fear.

The large majority of those with the virus have no symptoms. Next to that, are those with very minor symptoms. Then a tiny percentage experience more severe symptoms such as a cluster of breakouts and discharge when it surfaces, accompanied by feelings of nausea or fatigue.

The risks of catching the herpes virus are quite low when there are no symptoms, although it is possible. So, what if you are in a relationship or thinking of being in a relationship with someone who has very mild to no symptoms? The worst case scenario is that you could catch it from them. The good news is that contrary to popular belief, usually the physical symptoms are not life-changing. If they surface, they can be annoying or a minor inconvenience for the short time it occurs.

The most harmful thing about herpes is the fear and shame connected to it. Many doctors will not give you a herpes test without symptoms because they know since the majority of people have it, there's a good chance you will test positive and the fear and the shame you may experience will be far worse than the virus itself. The problem with this, is those with symptoms take the brunt of the stigma.

In the US and likely globally, close to 100% of people tested for herpes will test positive. This is because you've most likely been exposed to it at some point in your life. So, now you are anti-body positive, even though you have absolutely no symptoms, probably never will and are not contagious. The positive test results tend to send a person into a pit of emotions, including shame due to the stigma surrounding herpes.

In the 1970s the medical community differentiated between herpes simplex virus 1 and 2, for the first time creating the mindset that there is a "good" and "bad" virus. Basically, if you have one on your mouth you did nothing bad. I suspect this is because it is common for small children to extract the virus through kissing a relative, whereas the simplex 2 virus is only caught through sexual contact.

The pharmaceutical company, Burroughs Wellcome Co. created a huge advertising campaign promoting a new drug called Zovirax, opening up a new booming business for them, using fear as a huge aspect of their marketing campaign. Up until this point, herpes hadn't been much of an issue. Herpes simplex 2 has been around for about 1.6 million years. Science says simplex 1 has been around even longer, passed around by apes before they evolved into humans.

In 1982, Time Magazine ran a cover story about herpes titled, "The New Scarlet Letter." Authors of this article, John Leo and Maureen Dowd reinforced the stigma around herpes and through their judgment of the sexual revolution they referred to herpes as putting an end the sexual revolution as if it were some kind of punishment. This article resulted in thousands of sufferers going into months of depression and self-shame. The article insinuated those who are infected with the virus were dirty people with low morals—a true example of sex shaming. This was irresponsible journalism and yet these narratives are still being played out in today's media.

It is time for the lie around herpes to stop. It's a very manageable virus and for the vast majority who do have symptoms, no more inconvenient than a temporary pimple or a mosquito bite.

It is time that herpes is eliminated from entertainment media and comedians' routines. Don't they realize that by making herpes jokes they are laughing at and shaming close to 70% of their audience? There is no other infection that exists where those with it, are shamed and made fun of because of it. There is so much fear associated with it, yet the symptoms are not life-threatening, usually non-existent or very minor.

The only time there is a great risk, is when a woman is infected late in pregnancy. If a herpes outbreak is present when it is time to give birth, a cesarean section will protect the child. If a woman had the virus before pregnancy or was infected early in the pregnancy, the chance that her baby will be infected is less than 1%.

Herpes is the most misunderstood, misinformed, overreacted to virus in existence. We all have a responsibility to be compassionate on this topic. Be compassionate toward those infected. Be compassionate toward those who aren't and have bought into the fear and over dramatization around it.

If you have herpes and are about to be with a new lover and fear being rejected, take a breath, be honest and disclose. If they can't handle it, the sooner you know the better. There's a good chance they have it too and are trying to figure out how to tell you. Maybe they have been with someone who had it and they understand the reality of it and are ok with it. It's better that you come forward with it now, than wait for a breakout and tell them after you are already in the relationship. Disclosure is to protect both of you. Just because you have one strain of herpes, it does not mean you can't catch another. It's not just about protecting them but yourself as well.

If you don't have it and have developed feelings for someone who has and you're fearful... relax, especially if they have a mild case. Those infected, are usually more freaked out about passing it on than those who don't have it are about getting it. They will tell you when they know or believe they are contagious. Most couples in this situation experience sexually vibrant relationships with one person infected and the other never catching the virus.

For women with herpes, a wonderful website offers support, education, and compassion. It is PinkTent.com, created by founder, Dr. Kelly Martin Schuh. There is another website called HerpesOpportunity.com by founder Adrial Dale. These two I am familiar with through my own research, run by people with the virus and through their own experience, they are inspired to help others. You can also reach out to me for support at Jaitara.com.

As an energy healer, I am always looking out for the best ways to stay healthy and whole in the body, emotions, and soul. PEMF mats are groundbreaking in their ability to heal the body. They are Health Canada and FDA approved. Although claims of healing herpes cannot be made about the mats, I want to share about two amazing case studies.

I know a couple that had herpes. When they first got together, she had a very mild strain and he was one of the few with a much stronger strain. She caught his strain and was shocked by the severity of the symptoms compared to what she was used to. They purchased a PEMF mat. They used the mat daily and within a short time, neither of them experienced a herpes symptom again. That was over six years ago, and they are still symptom-free. When they looked back upon their life, the only thing they had done differently was the mat. A healthy diet and living a low-stress life are important to keeping symptoms at a minimum, which they were already doing.

What others experience with these mats is nothing short of a miracle. Many who have had pain in their body for years have their pain disappear in as fast as one session. People with Parkinson's, are having their symptoms stop. If you want to know more, you can connect with me at Jaitara.com/Store

4. ASKING FOR WHAT YOU WANT:

It is common for the feminine to hold back and have difficulty speaking into what she wants sexually. When this happens, her nurturing nature does not want to hurt the feelings of her masculine partner and have him think he is not pleasing her, even when it's true. Her priority is emotional connection. She may find it easier to be less sexually fulfilled than to communicate with him to touch her differently than he is. Also, when in the heat of the moment, she does not want to break the flow, so she will go with the flow, even if it's not flowing the way she secretly desires.

I've met many women who struggle with this. I was one for many years. I wanted so much for the words to come out and communicate more of what I wanted during sex, but my voice stayed silent. Every time, it was out of concern for hurting my partner's feelings, or out of concern that I was taking too long to orgasm, so I faked it, so he would feel good as a lover. I was in my forties before I grew out of this.

If you recognize yourself in this scenario, it's time to claim your voice. Trust me, your partner wants to be the lover you desire. The healthy masculine wants to please the feminine. He wants to be her hero. He desires her happiness and her pleasure.

I recommend having this conversation outside of the bedroom, outside of the heat of the moment. If you are the feminine, share what you love about how he touches and pleasures you. Then share what is not working for you, what you would love him to do differently or something new you would like to try.

If you are the masculine and it feels like your partner is shy, inhibited or holding back in some way, then gently encourage her to open up and provide you guidance on how she wants to be touched. Patience is key here. Every woman's body is different in what feels good. Conscious communication, intuition, patience, and exploration are how to figure this out.

You will also communicate what you desire from her, but if she is shy or holding back with her communication, address that first. Otherwise through wanting to please you, she is likely to sacrifice her desires for yours. Remember many women need to learn how to receive. Hold space for her by giving to her first and she will reciprocate your desires with greater enthusiasm.

When I work privately with couples, I guide them through a communication process in the form of a dyad, where both partners feel fully heard, seen and honored by one another and open to a new awareness, pleasure and discovery in their relationship. I guide them on new ways to touch one another through massage, while communicating what works, what doesn't, and what they would like done differently.

We all have a Responsibility to speak up and communicate what we want, how we want to be approached and touched. Women desire to feel penetrated in their heart and soul by a man before he moves to penetrate her yoni. This is a learned art and skill and one not commonly taught. It can also evolve with maturity.

If you are a teen or young adult, you can be fully present as a healthy mature masculine or healthy mature feminine by listening to your own heart, by paying attention to what feels right in your gut and honoring one another's boundaries. Connect with one another through eye contact and communicate with sensitivity to one another's vulnerability.

Speaking up and asking for what you want doesn't only apply to new partners. I've worked with couples where the woman was in emotional pain she had been hiding from her husband because she did not know how to ask for what she wants sexually. When there is a lack of communication at the beginning of the relationship, the longer it goes unaddressed, the more challenging it is for her to speak up. The woman will fear that her Beloved's feelings will be hurt even more as more time passes. As time passes she feels she can't possibly let him know that he has not been her ideal lover for so long, so to protect his feelings, she stays silent.

I once worked with a couple married thirty years. She was in painful frustration due to feeling unfulfilled sexually. She had never learned to ask for what she wants. Her husband believed by her lack of speaking up that she was content. By bringing me in as their guide, I helped them to open their communication while keeping feelings and egos intact. He was very responsive in learning how to give to her in new ways, and she was finally able to communicate and guide him on what felt good to her body so she could experience the pleasure she desired.

Although the intention behind her silence was based on compassion, her choice to stay silent for so long was not the most enlightened choice. Fortunately, she took the steps to shift this by bringing me in to help.

A good clue to know if a lover is holding back on communicating their sexual desires is if they do not speak into them. No matter how good of a lover you are, there is always something unique about each partner for us to learn about and something new to explore.

Some experienced lovers are highly intuitive and true artists. They know how to open you to deeper depths of pleasure and ecstasy by being attentive to response, the breath, eye contact, and body language. They know how to penetrate the very core of your being, as you explode one another's souls into light and blissful euphoria. This may be you. Yay! Sending you a high five!

Everyone can learn to be such an artist. If you've been together for a long time, learning every fragment and nuance of one another's bodies adds another layer of brilliance to your artistry. Even so, it's still a good idea to check in. Even if you've been married for years, you can still be surprised by the new discoveries that can unfold.

VOICE AND VISIBILITY
*"When you hold back to protect vulnerability within your
Sexual Energy, you are holding back… period!
This reflects in your Voice, your Presence
and diminishes your Visibility.
Own your power with grace.
BE You, so we can SEE You."*
~ *Sacred Sexual Enlightenment Wisdom Cards*

5. *SUPPORTIVE LANGUAGE:*

When in a love relationship, it is so important to be supportive in a way that helps one another continue to grow to be the best you can be. The masculine will grow through challenge. The feminine will grow through praise. It is imperative to understand this with intimate relationships, and it also applies to friends, family members, and professional relationships.

As boys, the masculine will say things like, "I bet you can't do this… ," and it will challenge them to do that thing. Men who are predominantly masculine know they like to be challenged to move forward in their life. In the business world, men love the challenge of competition. So, with challenge being what works for the masculine, it's common to make the mistake of trying to support their feminine partner by challenging her. This does not work. In fact, it has the reverse effect.

The feminine grows by praise. The masculine must never hold back in his praise of the feminine to support her growth. Whatever quality is being praised, that is the quality that will magnify within her.

Once I was with a lover and as he stood behind me, gazing at me with awe and admiration, he said with such feeling, "You have such a beautiful ass." My response was to work out even more to greater enhance the shape of my butt.

So, if you are a man and you want to see more of your woman's radiance, tell her she is radiant. If you'd like her to exercise more, tell her how much you love her body. If you want her to open up to you more sexually, penetrate her heart and soul, and as you do, tell her how radiant she is and how she fills up your heart when she opens to you in this way.

If you are a woman, challenging your man does not mean being combative with him or putting up obstacles he has to get past. Coming from kindness and compassion is key with any communication. If there is a trait you want to see in him, tell him what kind of traits you admire in a man. That will challenge him to be that man for you.

The masculine loves freedom. Give him space. Love your own life and live it without making him the center of your universe. This will challenge him by wanting to work at keeping you in his life.

To be supportive and help one another grow, be Responsible and supportive with your language. Whether you are offering praise to the feminine or challenging the masculine, do so with an open heart, through love, respect, and kindness. One of *The Four Agreements* by Don Miguel Ruiz is to be impeccable with your word. This is about being impeccable with your word and being aware of the different languages that the feminine and masculine respond to.

In the workplace, this can be very effective. Competition and challenge results in a woman having to go further into her masculine to keep up. That can be exhausting for her. When a business environment includes a lot of praise, expressing appreciation for the team, the women are especially inspired to do much more for the company.

6. PROFESSIONAL VOICE:

If you are a professional coach, healer, speaker, therapist or bodywork practitioner and you work in the field of sexuality, you have a great Responsibility to do whatever inner work, research, and training is necessary to serve from the highest place of integrity. This should go without saying, however, I have witnessed this being misaligned and it always makes me cringe. That said, I acknowledge that I am Responsible for my own feelings and reactivity.

If you are seeking the work of a professional who works in the field of sexuality, whether it is to learn about sacred sexuality, to receive emotional healing around sexual wounding or to spice up your sex life, you have a Responsibility to yourself to do your own research.

Back in 2012, I was connected to a woman on Facebook. We've never met in person. I discovered her through a search I did when I was looking for some business coaching. I liked her energy and the way she taught marketing. A few years later she came forward announcing herself as a sexual healer. She shared with me she had just spent twenty years healing her own sexual wounds and that she recently had a breakthrough and decided to help others with what had worked for her. That's wonderful. Most of the knowledge and wisdom I have is from my own personal journey.

What felt misaligned and out of integrity to me is that she was promoting herself as having twenty years of experience as a master sexual healer. This was very misleading. I knew from following her work for three years and from what she shared with me, this was a brand-new career focus and I'm sure she had no professional training as a healer. Working on your own personal healing for twenty years and working professionally with clients are two very different realities.

Dealing with sexual trauma is deep work and can go to some very dark places unimaginable for many. My life experience with my own sexual healing and my spiritual journey surrounding that, is a huge asset to my abilities as a professional. Yet, life experience on its own is not enough.

There are many things that can come up when working with emotional trauma you must be prepared for and knowledgeable in dealing with. It's the combination of my life experience, plus years of professional training, emotional healing experience, and practice that contributes to my ability to care for my clients, no matter what may come up.

Recently I spoke with a women's circle facilitator who shared that she wanted to expand into teaching around Sacred Sexuality and asked what books I can recommend. I smiled and recommended this one and let her know it would be coming out soon. However, I hope she was planning to prepare herself beyond just reading.

Reading books alone does not qualify you to teach such a deep and delicate topic as sexuality. If you are a professional, wanting to expand your practice into the realm of sexuality, whether it's to help women feel more sensual in their bodies, or to dive into emotional healing work for both men and women, be in integrity and get the best training possible so you are well prepared to handle hidden trauma if it surfaces in your workshop space.

A sex therapist is trained in the physiological processes of human sexuality. They work collaboratively with physicians to address the entire causes of sexual concerns including all the layers of biology. They can also work as a marriage counselor, psychologist or clinical social worker. Except for sexual surrogate therapists, their work is primarily talk therapy.

Whether you're seeking a sex therapist, emotional healer who specializes in sexuality, intimacy coach, Sacred Sexuality mentor, or Tantra facilitator, do your research. If they do not have training listed on their website, or their marketing materials, ask them how many years' experience they've had actually working with clients. Get a referral. Ask what training they've received. Look for client testimonials. Be Responsible to yourself by asking the right questions and by doing your research.

RESPONSIBILITY OF CONSENT

I know for most reading this book, I am speaking into the obvious. Consent is such an important a topic. If you are a teen or young adult, new to sexual activity, it's especially important for you to understand what true consent really is.

If you are a parent, I recommend you pass on this information to your teen.

The only communication that is a consensual "yes" is an eye contact, "yes." "No" does not mean "if you pressure me enough or coerce me enough, I may say maybe or yes." It means "no."

"Maybe" does not mean "yes." It means "no." "Yes" without eye contact means "no." When the person is saying yes but cannot look you in the eye and instead is looking downward or away from you, they are really saying something like, "I really don't want to, but I really want you to like me so I'll do it just so that you will like me."

The only "yes" that means "yes," is an enthusiastic direct eye contact "yes," period! Anything less than that, they are not ready. If you try to sweet talk them into sex or convince them in any way, you are abusing your power over them and manipulating them into doing something they really do not want to do.

You do not want someone agreeing to have sex for the sake of going along with it. You want them to really want you. You want to feel their desire emanating from their being. A true "yes" is not just the speaking of the word "yes." The only true "yes" is when you hear and feel an enthusiastic ecstatic "YES, YES!", otherwise, you are still getting a "no."

There is a wonderful YouTube video titled, *Tea and Consent*, where they use offering someone a cup of tea as a metaphor for getting consent to have sex. It's quite humorous and really puts things into perspective. I highly recommend you view it. I especially love the original British version. They also have one with an American English narration as well. If you are a parent, show it to your teen. You may prefer the British version, as the American version uses more explicit language.

It's simple really, you would not try to coerce someone into having a cup of tea. If you ask and they say no thanks, you accept that. To do otherwise is just silly. You also would not assume that just because they wanted tea yesterday, they want tea today. You would not try to wake someone up who is sleeping to give them a cup of tea and you would especially not try to pour the tea down their throat. There are many more examples in this video, which show the ridiculousness of trying to make someone drink tea when they do not want tea. Sex is no different.

Girls who do not have a strong father role model in their life and have not received the father love or guidance they need, are especially vulnerable to coercion. Saying "no" can be difficult for them. They want so much to be accepted. This I know well, as I was one of those teens. In my youth I had sex usually because I wanted to feel loved, not because I felt ready for sex.

I was in my forties before I learned how to say "no" as a complete sentence. I thought I had to explain my "no," justify it or was uncomfortable that my "no" may hurt the feelings of another, even if they were a complete stranger. This is very common among many girls and women.

I am focusing on the importance of boys and men receiving consent from the feminine because we generally think of receiving consent as applying to the masculine. Usually, it does, as it's the nature of the masculine to take the lead. However, there are exceptions; girls and women are sometimes the pursuers. Receiving consent is mandatory no matter who is taking the lead. Teen boys are also vulnerable. How they are seen in the eyes of others can be very important to them. If they agree to sex before they are ready, the sexual connection is misaligned and can come with consequences.

Be aware, be in integrity and be kind to one another. Sex is too beautiful, too special and too powerful to enter into it prematurely. You are too worthy and precious to give your body to another unless the timing feels absolutely perfect. To honor this in yourself and in your potential partner is an enlightened choice.

RESPONSIBILITY OF DISCERNMENT

"You CANNOT unfuck someone.

So before crossing the point of no return and risking the potential messiness, confusion, feelings of regret and wounding that can ensue following a less than conscious or less than enthusiastically chosen sexual union:

Connect with yourself and feel into what's most important and true.

Be sure other has connected with their self and has felt into what's most important and true.

Connect with each other about what's most important and true".

~ Anthony Lemme; Trauma Specialist

BE DISCERNING with both the timing and with whom you share yourself with. Sexual energy is exceptionally powerful. When we have sex with another, we are interlocking our bodies and literally merging our energy fields.

When I was an active member of the Well Being Ministry at the Agape International Spiritual Center near Los Angeles, there was a day when one of the practitioners brought in her aura video camera. This camera takes a video of the energy field that surrounds your body. It actually photographs and videotapes the colors and movement of your auric field. When one of us was lying on the massage table, we could see the aura of that person. Then when the healing practitioner stepped in, we could see their energy field moving around them. When they placed their hands on the person on the table, both of their auric fields merged and shifted in colors and structure.

So, imagine what happens to the energy field during intercourse, when a man is literally inside the body of a woman, activating the most powerful human energy force… the sexual life force. With a same sex relationship, bodies are also merging. The merging of energy is powerful whether physical penetration is taking place or not. Imagine how the other person impacts the actual structure of your energy field. This is why it is so important to be discerning.

You may be considering sharing yourself with someone new who is a good hearted person but maybe they have issues in their life they are working through and have heaviness or blocks in their energy. Think carefully before you merge your body with theirs. You may want to wait until they have worked things through and created a shift. Wait for when their energy is raised to a higher frequency.

In the meantime, if you want to be there for them, you can comfort them through friendship and with hugs.

Each of us is a powerful energy force with a direct impact on whom we share our energy with, and our sexual partner's energy directly affects us. Be Responsible with your own power and be Responsible through discernment.

RESPONSIBILITY OF LIFESTYLE COMPATIBILITY

Being in integrity with compatibility in relation to your lifestyle preference will save you from a lot of heartache, confusion, and frustration. This may involve a bit of soul searching and experimentation to get clear on what your lifestyle preference really is. Be honest with yourself and be honest with your partner and potential partners.

Those who live a polyamory or non-monogamous lifestyle in integrity and truth, can experience an abundance of love in their relationships with multiple partners. It's rare, but when lovers are able to successfully live a full-time polyamory lifestyle, it can be quite beautiful.

I've seen the word polyamory misused often. I've seen people say they are polyamorous, but really, they are just promiscuous or living a swinger's lifestyle. So, what's the difference? Translated, the word polyamory means "multiple loves" — "loves" being the key word here. It does not mean to have sex with multiple people. Yes, having sex is an aspect of this lifestyle, but true polyamory is when there it is a multiple love relationship. It is when there is a genuine heart connection with everyone involved. It may not mean that all partners are deeply in love with one another, but there is a special bond, and an honoring of a heart connection. For this to work, all parties must know about one another, be in full agreement, truth and ensure everyone's boundaries being 100% respected.

Often, but not always, there is a primary relationship such as a spouse, then new intimate partners come in. Done with integrity, a new partner only enters the relationship circle through discussion with the primary partner and others involved, and all are in full agreement that the new partner enters the relationship. This requires maturity and a level of personal growth, confidence and a belief system that does not come naturally to many people. I know some who live this lifestyle and do it very well.

If you are bouncing around having sex with a variety of people, with no emotional involvement or connection, that's promiscuity, not polyamory. If that makes you happy and you are not hurting anyone, then all is well. Connect with your body sensations, thoughts and feelings around this. If it is not bringing you joy, then perhaps take a deeper look within. If it feels more like an addiction then I urge you to seek support from a sex addict professional.

If you are in a committed relationship and you have sex with others without your partner knowing, that is infidelity, not polyamory. It's only non-monogamy or polyamory when there is a genuine connection with everyone involved and all parties are aware and in full agreement.

Swinging is when couples engage in partner swapping. This is a lifestyle where often the couple will host a private party in their home and invite other couples and singles to participate in an open sex party. When practiced with integrity, there are strict rules in place, such as "no" means no, there is full disclosure of STIs, and condoms are provided.

A swinger's lifestyle is primarily about having multiple sexual partners without necessarily a love connection, other than the couples with one another. Singles also participate in this type of lifestyle. Usually, only single women can attend a party solo, and single men must be accompanied by a woman. This is to maintain a feeling of safety for the women and to keep the gender quota balanced.

If you want to live a polyamorous lifestyle, you must be with a partner who also wants to live a polyamorous lifestyle, or it will not work. If you know you are monogamous, and you agree to try swinging or polyamory with your partner just to make them happy but you're not really into it, you are setting yourself up for heartache and misalignment in your relationship. You are being out of integrity with yourself and with them. If you are monogamous and feel coerced by your partner to try a swinger or polyamorous lifestyle, it is unfair to you and it dishonors your boundaries.

If you are in a relationship and one of you is determined to explore an alternative lifestyle of polyamory or swinging and the other doesn't, I suggest these three choices:

- You terminate the relationship.
- You agree to honor your individual preferences for a short trial period, with the monogamous partner staying true to their preference while

giving the other partner space to explore. Then after the agreed time, you decide what your agreements will be moving forward by honoring what is true for each of you. This option can be quite challenging for the monogamous partner, but it can work.
- If your desire to stay with your partner is stronger than your desire to explore this new lifestyle, you honor the boundaries of the monogamous partner. Keep it as a fantasy but do not pursue it as a reality.

Perhaps a good alternative is to try role playing and pretend to be different people. As long as this is alluring and exciting for both parties involved, you can have fun with it. Discuss new explorations you can play with that appeal to both of you. Focus on your gratitude for the beautiful love and connection you share. Savor that. Nurture that. Bask in the beauty of this precious love you cherish together.

If you are monogamous and you enter into a relationship with someone who is non-monogamous or a swinger, enter the relationship from a space of acceptance. If you go into it thinking that if you love them enough they will change for you, you're setting yourself up for a painful reality. Accepting such an arrangement can be challenging or it can be an opportunity for self-growth. There is no right or wrong here, simply the Responsibility to be honest with you and to do what is true for you.

RESPONSIBILITY OF BODY AWARENESS

You have a Responsibility to know your own sexual body, and your partner's. There are specific biological facts that by being familiar with them, you can be a better lover for yourself and your partner. The following are a few examples of information about men and women's sexual bodies that may not be common knowledge that all men and women can benefit from knowing.

1. MEN'S BODIES:

Did you know that men also have a G-spot? It's very much like the shape and size of the female G-spot. It's the prostate. Massaged properly, a man can experience an orgasm from the stimulation of his prostate alone, just as a woman can experience a G-spot orgasm. A female partner can help him with this most effectively by wearing surgical gloves, so the fingernails do not scratch or tear the delicate skin of his prostate. Some men love this type of stimulation. Some are very uncomfortable with it, as it involves anal penetration. Some women are comfortable giving a prostate massage, and some are not. Be true to what feels good for you as both giver and receiver. The prostate can also be massaged on the exterior of the body by applying pressure on the perineum.

Massaging the prostate is not only pleasurable for many men, but it is very healthy for the prostate and helps prevent it from becoming enlarged. A man can learn to massage his own prostrate by contracting the pubococcygeus muscles, also known as the PC muscles. These are the same muscles you squeeze to stop yourself from going pee. Both men and women have PC muscles.

All life is a miracle of creation and our bodies are perfectly designed with clear intention. The pleasure and health benefit a man receives from prostate stimulation is part of his Divine Design, or it would not be possible. Accept it. Embrace it. And proceed in whatever method both you and your partner feel comfortable with. Remember, self-massage through exercising the PC muscles is a great option.

By contracting the PC muscles, combined with specific breath techniques, a man can eliminate premature ejaculation issues and learn to last much longer during sex. I have taught this to men who suffered from premature ejaculation and have witnessed some of them cry tears of joy as they learn how to control their energy for the first time.

When practicing this same technique regularly, a man can experience multiple orgasms without ejaculation. A world expert on Tao Sexuality, Mantak Chia goes into great detail on this technique in his bestselling book, *The Multi-Orgasmic Man*.

2. WOMEN'S BODIES:

In the Chapter *The Gift*, I shared about the ligaments near the opening of the vagina and how when these ligaments do not relax properly before intercourse, they can be damaged. I also shared how these ligaments around the vagina support the bladder and rectum, so anything that damages the vaginal structure can also damage the bladder and rectum.

Entering a woman's vagina must not be rushed. Contrary to what many of the sex scenes depict in movies and on TV shows, women do not like being rushed to intercourse. Women require time to warm up, for bodily fluids to be produced, for her muscles and ligaments to be relaxed and for her yoni to swell to where she is physically ready to receive a man inside her. Most women cannot orgasm from penetration alone. They require clitoral stimulation to reach orgasm.

When intercourse happens quickly, the body language and response of the feminine can send mixed signals to the masculine partner. He's thinking, "She loves this!" and maybe she does. But, she may also feel that more foreplay would be preferable. Taking Responsibility for communication is key here. If you didn't know before, you now know there is a health risk involved with entering into intercourse too soon before a woman's body is prepared.

Most of the time a woman prefers to be savored with kisses and be caressed all over her body before intercourse. At times variation can add spice to the mix. When caught up in the throes of passion, being ravished quickly and passionately can be incredible, hot and exciting. Savoring first, then diving in with primal abandon is often a lovely combination. Connect with your partner and be aware of what is desired in heat of the moment.

There are twelve different types of orgasms that women can experience. Some can be powerful, others are much more subtle and smaller in intensity.

· · ·

THEY ARE:

- Clitoral
- G-Spot
- Kissing on the mouth
- Anal
- Multiple
- Blend of multiple points simultaneously
- A-Spot – deep inside the vagina toward the belly button
- Cervical
- Nipple stimulated
- Mental
- Urethra
- Zonegasm on typically non-sexual areas of the body

For a more detailed explanation, simply Google: *Twelve different types of female orgasm*. Have fun with your research!

According to sex educator Lucia Paxton, the orgasm is when your body reaches the relaxed state just before climax. The climax is the peak that occurs when a woman experiences a few seconds of pelvic floor muscle contractions. Through clitoral stimulation, a woman can build her orgasmic energy and remain in an extended orgasm as long as she wants, once she knows how.

The Honor Society of Nursing states, *"An orgasm is the climax of sexual arousal, or the release of built-up sexual tension that's felt throughout the body."*

According to various articles and resources, an orgasm is the highest peak of sexual pleasure. *Climax* is used to describe this because it means *a peak*, however a sexual climax and an orgasm are one in the same.

Personally, I've always referred to my climax as an orgasm, and my extended orgasm, as being orgasmic. I also love referring to it as an expanded orgasm, as when I am in that state, I am in a state of expansion. I researched to find the correct wording for this book. Based on the information I just shared with you, I choose the word "orgasm" when referring to the peak of sexual release, simply because I love the word and because it's the one most commonly used. In my sexual enlightenment programs, being in an expanded orgasmic state is an aspect of my teaching and the practice of *Orgasmic Creation*, which I write about in the next chapter.

3. MEN AND WOMEN:

Men and women's bodies are dramatically different from one another, not just in appearance but in our sexual response. Men reach orgasm far more easily than women, on purpose… for procreation. Not only do most women not reach orgasm during intercourse, but a very large percentage of straight women do not orgasm when with a partner at all.

Chapman University did a survey on 52,000 people to discover who is more likely to orgasm with a partner. These were people of various sexual orientations. In this study, they discovered that heterosexual men had the highest rate of success, whereas heterosexual women had the lowest percentage of success achieving orgasm with a partner.

. . .

HERE ARE THE RESULTS:

- Heterosexual men 95%
- Lesbian women 86%
- Gay men 89%
- Bisexual men 88%
- Bisexual women 66%
- Heterosexual women 65%

They discovered that the three sex acts that create the highest possibility for women to achieve orgasm are deep kissing, genital stimulation, and oral sex. When all three of these are applied the chances are the best.

In this survey, 30% of men believed that vaginal intercourse is the best way for a woman to achieve orgasm, while only 35% of the heterosexual women actually achieved orgasm from just intercourse. Meanwhile, 80% of straight women and 91% of lesbian women achieved orgasm by combining all three; deep kissing, genital stimulation, and oral sex. Women love oral sex because it feels really beautiful and it works.

Women, on average, take fifteen to twenty minutes to reach orgasm. Men take on average less than five minutes. The oxytocin hormone is released when orgasm takes place. When a woman gets a surge of oxytocin it energizes her. When a man gets a surge of oxytocin, their testosterone levels plummet and they get sleepy. All very valid facts on why it makes the most sense for a man to pleasure the woman first.

Women take longer and last longer. So, after orgasm they still have lots of energy to keep going for the man.

Whereas if the man ejaculates before she is fulfilled, there is a good chance he may fall asleep leaving her unfulfilled. Also, for many women, once they've experienced clitoral orgasm, it's much easier to achieve another one through intercourse because she is already activated, so you can still experience the beauty of reaching orgasm together.

For the best sex for everyone involved, the man must give to the woman first. Kiss her deeply and give oral sex or be very skilled with your hands… or give oral sex. Continue expressing your full unbridled passion together, giving, sharing, merging together, devouring one another, basking in the ecstatic messiness.

I've given you a few examples of how you can be more aware of your own body and the other's and how that supports deeper connection, pleasure, and wellbeing. I've given you a few tidbits of techniques to encourage you to do more research, educate yourself and openly communicate with your partner.

There is an abundance of knowledge available online. This is not a how to have sex book, as much as it is a guide to remind you who you are as a Divine being, how your primal sexual body merges with your spirit body, to encourage you to explore enlightened sexuality and how to live a joyful radiant love life with or without a partner, through healing, awareness and expression.

WELL-BEING

Well-Being of our physical body, spirit body, emotional body and energy body is necessary to experience a life of pleasure.
This card is a reminder to feed all your bodies.

Feed your Physical Body healthy organic foods, exercise, fresh air and loving touch.

Feed your Emotional Body by healing the past, to enjoy the deliciousness of the present.

Feed your Spirit Body meditation and prayer.

Feed your Energy Body by breathing deeply. Learn about your Chakras. Keep them activated, vibrant and open.

One body influences the other. They are all connected. Love and nourish them to savor a life of Wellness and Pleasure.

4. ENERGETIC BODY:

If you are not familiar with the chakra system, it will serve you to do some research. Energetically, everything in our body is connected. If there is a contraction or block in energy flow in the 2nd chakra, it will also affect the flow of the other chakras, like a stone in the water creates ripples.

There is an abundance of information in books and on the Internet on the chakra system. Our bodies are magnificent miracles of creation and everything works together. Your body is the instrument you were born with. Learn how to be a maestro with your instrument.

Take responsibility for learning about your body's energetic system. When you carry emotional residue, it creates a block in your energy. E-motion is energy in motion. Take responsibility to keep your energy body clean and open. Explore it, heal it, understand it, love it, be compassionate with it, respect it and it will reveal new realms of power and bliss to you.

RESPONSIBILITY OF REFLECTION

The world that surrounds each of us is a reflection of who we are. We are powerful creators. I know this sounds cliché but we do create our own reality, even the stuff in our life we do not like or want. If something or someone exists in your life that is unpleasant, reflect within to see what you have been focusing on to attract that. The stronger the emotional charge is around what you focus on, the more it will show up.

For years until my early forties, I attracted misaligned partners. In my mid-thirties, I had a partner who would get drunk every Friday, spending all his party money with his buddies. Saturday was our date night. Every Saturday I'd end up with a hung-over, broke date and I had to foot the bill.

The next partner I ended up with drank too much and was verbally abusive. After him, I ended up with a partner who drank too much and was extremely verbally abusive. I have never been much of a drinker. I could probably count the number of times I've actually been drunk in my lifetime on one hand and that hasn't happened in over thirty years. It's just never felt like fun, yet I created a reality where I consistently ended up in intimate relationships with drinkers. My lack of self-worth at the time started it. Staying in that same pattern continued it.

With each partner, it seemed to get worse. Each was more intensified in what I did not want from the last. I finally recognized this was my creation, my dream; that I had to make a shift within me if I wanted to attract a healthier more aligned man into my life and to live a dream that felt good to me. So, I took a break from being in relationships, did some soul searching and worked on me. I discovered Reiki and became a certified Reiki Master Teacher. I'm sure learning the energy healing practice of Reiki played a large role in the shift I created in my energy field.

The next man who came into my life was a light social drinker and verbal abuse was not an aspect of his character.

He was mature, interesting and honoring. It was healing simply being in his presence. Within two months of meeting him, I had my day of the Grackle experience that forever shifted the direction of my life.

He was a wonderful lover and will always be a dear friend. We were lovers for fourteen years. I have embraced our friendship as one of my most beautiful creations. His presence in my life has played an integral role in how I matured as a woman.

Once I took Responsibility for my own reflection and explored what needed to shift within me, I created a shift in the world around me. As I healed the emotional residue around my sexual wounding and explored my connection between God and my sexual body, my reflection changed into something new, beautiful and beyond my imagination.

Taking Responsibility for your reflection is a lifelong practice. Challenges are part of life. There will always be contrast. It's how we move through the contrast, expand from it, learn from it, gain clarity from it and become wiser from it that makes the difference in our happiness.

The contrast in your life is a blessing and a gift giving you clarity on what you don't want, so you can more powerfully create what you do want. Observe your reflection. Do you like it? Are you happy with the reality that surrounds you and those in it? If so, what a blessing it is! If not, what a blessing it is!

Is there someone who triggers you? A trigger is when you experience reactivity versus response to another's presence, words or actions. A trigger occurs when someone is mirroring an aspect of you that is misaligned. Otherwise, you would not feel triggered. You would simply observe their behavior and respond accordingly. A trigger is a blessing in how it alerts you to look within, heal, expand and shift to a more aware, aligned and wiser you.

How we do one thing is how we do everything. My reflection shifted into something much more appealing to me when I started doing my inner sexual healing work and focused on spiritual growth.

Only you are Responsible for your reflection. If you don't like it then explore why. Are there emotional wounds you haven't healed? Is there something or someone you are not at peace with? Do you feel a disconnect between your spirit body and sexual body? The answers to these questions are gems and blessings for you to create a new reflection of greater joy and pleasure for you.

RESPONSIBILITY OF ACCEPTANCE

We all have a Responsibility to be accepting of other people's choices without judgment. If you are reading this book, you are most likely on a spiritual path. Some people are not on a spiritual path and content to simply engage in primarily primal sex. They may be in a loving relationship or single but including spirituality into the mix is just not their thing.

Some people have sexual fetishes that may seem weird or even distorted from your perspective. As long as they are not hurting others and are consenting adults then it is no one's place to judge. If they are hurting themselves in some way, you can send them love and wish they find the peace and help they need, or reach out to help, or compassionately detach.

The world is comprised of much diversity. In the Vedic teachings, the only rule is to never intentionally harm another. As long as this rule is in place, we have a Responsibility to not judge, no matter how weird another's choices or lifestyle may seem to us. Accept them for who they are. Focus on you. Do what brings joy to you and those who agree with your point of view will show up in your life.

The science of Ayurveda teaches there are three primary body types: Kapha, Pitta, and Vata. Most people have a primary body type, then a secondary and a third. It's also possible to be a balance of all three. When you put together all the possibilities of combinations, there are ten body types that humans have. Kaphas are naturally round or curvy. Vatas have naturally slim and slender bodies, and Pittas have naturally muscular bodies.

I am primarily Kapha with Pitta as a strong secondary. My upper body is more muscular and tones faster than my lower body when I work out. My lower body is round and plump even when I work out. I will never be slim and slender like the Vata because it is not how I was born. There was a time in my past when I wanted to be and went on starvation diets trying. Then I learned to love and adore my voluptuousness.

Kaphas gain weight the easiest. A Kapha is happiest when they learn to find pleasure in the extra softness and plumpness of their body. Having a healthy body is what's most important and beautiful regardless of size and shape.
We have a Responsibility to ourselves to be accepting of our own bodies. I've seen too many get caught up in the

pain and stress of trying to make their body something it will never be. A Kapha will never be a Vata and vice versa. Love your body as it is. If getting more fit is a desire, do so from a space of love. This also sets a positive role model for the younger generation.

I developed a process titled, the *Sacred Lover Body Types*™ to help others love the body they are in. This is based on the science of Ayurveda. Each of the *Sacred Lover Body Types*™ has gifts and challenges. Some body types are more naturally compatible with some than with others. Each body type has specific character traits. You can actually tell by a person's body type and body language what some of their sexual expression preferences are.

If you want to discover your *Sacred Lover Body Types*™, go to Jaitara.com/Store to receive the free assessment and video.

RESPONSIBILITY OF POWER

1. PERSONAL POWER:

We are all powerful beings. I know from experience what it means to be at the receiving end of misaligned personal power. At age sixteen, my boyfriend abused his power as he manipulated my heart, lured me into believing I was in love, so he could become my pimp and control me through my love. After I freed myself from him, a woman abused her power as she became my pimp and controlled me through fear by threatening to beat me if I did not do as she said. These are extreme examples, but any form of manipulation or control over another is abusive behavior. It can be a source of intense emotional pain and wounding, especially when inflicted upon a sexual relationship. Be aware and protect yourself. Seek help if you need to.

Other forms of misaligned personal power may not result in emotional wounding and only succeed when there is an agreement from both parties involved, even if this agreement is not made on a conscious level. An example of this is when someone uses the power of their physical beauty to manipulate or coerce another into giving them or doing something they want. A more conscious way would be to connect heart to heart and share with the other what you desire and why it means so much to you.

Another example is when a partner threatens to withhold sex from the other to get what they want, or they flaunt sex to get what they want as if it is a form of payment. If you are offering your sexual energy as a payoff in the form of a playful game occasionally, then that's not manipulation. It's just fun. However, if you know you have a tendency to manipulate in this way, look within. Do not judge it. Simply acknowledge it. There is likely an unresolved wound at the root of this behavior. Find that, heal it, release it, learn and grow from it.

2. PROFESSIONAL POWER:

At the time of writing this book, there is a lot of attention in the media about the abuse of power in Hollywood. The Harvey Weinstein scandal has made public the pervasive sexual harassment and abuse of women and men in the entertainment industry. Bill Cosby was recently sentenced to imprisonment for sexual abuse. This abuse of power is not unique to Hollywood. It is prevalent in various businesses, especially those where there is a hierarchy of authority or status.

As victims of abuse step forward and speak up, it makes it easier for more to do so. Those in a position of leadership have a Responsibility to be humble, compassionate and respectful with their power. Those who have been disrespected or abused have a Responsibility to speak up, no matter how scary it may be. By taking this step, it reinforces the power of your voice and your boundaries, and it protects prospective future victims from the perpetrator.

I've witnessed an abuse of professional power in the alternative healing community, where a practitioner has given a session to a client that involved deep emotional healing and then they pursue a sexual relationship with them. When working with a client, whether the client hired the facilitator or whether the healing work was offered as a gift, the client is in a vulnerable position.

When I was trained as a Holistic Rebirther, I took a vow I would never date or have sexual relations with a client. I vowed that if I was interested in someone who I have worked with, even if they only come for one session, that I will wait a full year before moving forward with the possibility being intimate.

When I hold space for a client in my Holistic Rebirthing sessions, deep emotional healing is taking place, most often much deeper than the client imagined. I enter into a space of mother love, to be there for them as needed. I cannot be a mother and a lover simultaneously. They honor me with their trust and I honor them as God Source before me. They open their emotional body with me to their most vulnerable state.

My sexual energy is powerful. It would be an abuse of my power to enter an intimate connection with such a client. We would not be on equal footing as partners. By that, I do not mean I am better than. It is about honoring the healer and recipient relationship. There is a powerful, alluring energy that a healing practitioner can have, especially when the recipient is in such a vulnerable state. I agreed to enter the relationship as their facilitator. Once the healing has begun, I must stay in integrity as a professional and be there for them, maintaining and honoring that agreement.

If a mutual attraction was established between us before our first session, I can give them a choice. They have a choice to date me and I'll refer them to someone else for their session, or have a session with me, but not both.

A few years ago, someone I know was doing energy healing in the home of a woman who had attended one of my workshops. She had met him through me. She shared with me that while in her home doing his work, he flirted with her and suggested that they connect with one another. She shared with me she found the situation very awkward. This was a mature woman and a very clear example of how difficult it is for many women to speak up and just say no. Deep down she didn't want to hurt his feelings, so she struggled to speak up. I shared with her to simply tell him straight out that, although she appreciates the work he has done, she is not interested in getting together.

This facilitator does amazing work and has a good heart, but he abused his power. When we spoke about it, it was clear he underestimated the power of his influence over others. He failed to separate his professional Responsibility from his personal desires and in doing so, his client felt uncomfortable with the situation. The personal connection he hoped for with her did not happen and he received no referrals for his work.

If you are a facilitator of emotional healing and you find yourself attracted to your client, acknowledge it. If the attraction is mutual, then decide if you still want them as a client or if you want to pursue a personal relationship with them. Make a decision, one or the other. Do you want a personal relationship or professional relationship? Choose one, not both. Be in integrity with your professional power.

3. MEDIA POWER:

The media has a Responsibility for its power and impact on the topic of sexuality. Even in today's world with the raising of consciousness happening, the media still fits into the old paradigm of the virgin or whore, good girl or bad girl, good boy or bad boy archetypes. There are exceptions with some of the more recent ads I am seeing on TV, where they show the actors reveling in ecstasy because they used the sponsor's condom or lubricant. Not that their bliss depends upon the product, but at least it's a positive portrayal of both women and men owning the joy of their pleasure. Dove has done campaigns where they portray women of various shapes sizes and colors as beautiful. These are good examples, but we still have a way to go.

As adults, we have the wisdom to be discerning. The youth's emotional health and well-being depend upon the environment and guidance they are exposed to. Whether a parent or not, it's the Responsibility of all adults to be healthy role models for the youth. It's the Responsibility of all adults to call out the media when they are out of integrity or to boycott their programs.

I did a lot of research on the impact of sexual content in the media. The various resources I found said pretty much the same thing. The following is a segment from an article posted by *Psychology Today* on August 13th, 2012, written by Carolyn C. Ross MD, M.P.H., titled *Overexposed and Under-Prepared: The Effects of Early Exposure to Sexual Content:*

"The media provides a type of sex education to young people. Media messages normalize early sexual experimentation and portray sex as casual, unprotected and consequence-free, encouraging sexual activity long before children are emotionally, socially or intellectually ready.

High-Risk Sex. The earlier a child is exposed to sexual content and has sex, the likelier they are to engage in high-risk sex. Research shows that children who have sex by age 13 are more likely to have multiple sexual partners, engage in frequent intercourse, have unprotected sex and use drugs or alcohol before sex. In a study by researcher Dr. Jennings Bryant, more than 66 percent of boys and 40 percent of girls reported wanting to try some of the sexual behaviors they saw in the media (and by high school, many had done so), which increases the risk of sexually transmitted diseases and unwanted pregnancies."

"In dreams begin responsibility" ~ W.B. Yeats

SUMMARY

You intuitively know if you need to be more Responsible with something I shared in this chapter or in an area I did not write about. Observe yourself, learn from the experience and create a shift.

Just because I write this book, I am not immune to my own humanness. I still mess up. Being sexually enlightened is not about rising above our humanness, it is about moving through it, learning, expanding and evolving from it; transcending pain to wisdom, and merging our divinity with our sexuality. It is about having clear mutual agreements, integrity, and honoring yourself and others. Sexual Enlightenment is not a destination. It's a magical ongoing journey of discovery, exploration, connection, messiness, awakened ecstasy and spiritual expansion.

APPLYING THE 3RD SACRED LAW TO THE WORKPLACE

Applying Responsibility to the workplace is self-explanatory. I respect your intelligence enough that I won't go into much detail on this one. It's simple, if you're a leader of a business, you are responsible for ensuring that the workplace feels safe and maintains a respectful environment free from sexual harassment or degradation. You also must lead by example.

CHAPTER 8

The Invitation

The 4th Sacred Law of Sexual Enlightenment is **THE INVITATION**
—Inviting God Source into the sexual experience.

INVITATION
"Invite the Lover Essence of God Source into your
Sexual experience with or without a partner.
Breathe the energy up to the Divine, while
grounding it into your Root Chakra, for more
euphoric orgasms and a deeper connection to Source.
It is how we are Designed."
~ Sacred Sexual Enlightenment Wisdom Cards

WHEN WE EXTEND Invitation to Divine Source to experience the ecstasy of our physical experience, we offer a precious gift that enriches and permeates on a multidimensional level.

SEX, GOD & YOU

You are pure love. You are life. That is the essence of you in the physical body. When you return to the Divine transcendental realm you return as nonphysical love intelligence. Love connects all of us. Love can never die therefore we never die. We are eternal. God is love. Your love is the aspect of you that is pure God Source Energy.

When I write the words, God, Divine, Spirit, Source or Creator, for me, they are all one and the same. Our connection to God is personal. Insert whatever word you relate to most.

Atma is a Sanskrit word that means essence/breath/soul. In the Vedic teachings, we are Atmas inhabiting a body temple while here on Earth. Atma also means "real self," "innermost essence." Atma is the essence of bliss. It is divinity. You are Atma. You enter into your body as Atma and you return to the transcendental realm as Atma.

In plain English, this means you are divinity. You are bliss. You are love. This is your real self, your soul, your innermost essence that never changes. Breath holds your essence in your physical body. The breath leaving your body is your Atma returning to the Divine realm, returning home.

When you communicate with Source through prayer or meditation, what do you say? What are your thoughts? What is your intention? Are you asking for guidance, expressing gratitude, praying for others, asking for more peace, love, health or prosperity? These are beautiful prayers and intentions.

Do you also take time to extend an Invitation to Source?

Do you pour energy into expressing and sharing your love with Source? Do you invite those in the Divine realm to connect with your love and orgasmic energy simply for the joy of it, the fun of it and so they can be at the receiving end of it? This is the beauty of *The Invitation*.

I have been practicing the Invitation in this way for many years and I continue to be in awe of the power, beauty, and bliss of it. Besides my sexual expression, I also practice the Invitation in my morning meditation, when I dine, when I dance, when I swim in the ocean, basically when I engage in any form of pleasure. I love the joy I feel when sharing the pleasure of being in a body with my Divine Team and opening verbal Invitation for them to enjoy the presence of it with me.

When we express and share our love for Source, whether it is in the stillness of meditation, or in the midst of sexual expression, the pleasure sensation in the body and soul always increases, and it is so healing.

The Invitation opens you to greater awakening and awareness. It is a raising of energy and consciousness that leads to a deeper connection with self, God and one another. This practice creates greater sexual, emotional and spiritual fulfillment with or without a partner. It creates a deeper sense of inner peace and infuses energy into that which we are creating in life.

I love referring to Source as "My Divine Team," as I can feel the presence of multiple loving Divine beings watching over me, guiding me, enjoying my life with me.

When I extend the Invitation during my morning meditation practice, expressing my love to my Divine Team, I feel energetic jolts in my heart center that feel like pure joy.

I call them heartgasms. It literally feels like an orgasm in my heart center. It's like my Divine Team is sending their love right back at me with a big energetic kiss in response to the love I send them. The Invitation is a potent way to not only share your love of God but also to receive it back so that you can feel it in your body. It is sheer joy for both you and for your Divine Team.

This Invitation is a gift offering to God. It is most often done without asking for anything in return. An exception would be when also offering your body as a channel for healing. In my healing practice, I invite Source to use my body as a channel to pour healing love into my client. When I do this, I also direct my love toward the client and silently say to my Divine Team, "Thank you. I love you."

I feel that love with all my heart and offer it to them. In return, I feel jolts of beautiful energy flowing through me. Sometimes at this moment, the client's body will jolt slightly in response to the energy surge. This is a beautiful confirmation that the Invitation, combined with the giving and sharing of love is reciprocated by Source, through a return of healing energy that feels like pure bliss.

God Source experiences the physical through us. Respect comes hand in hand with any love relationship. Although the love of Source is always with us, active participation in our sexual experience requires Invitation. When we share our sexual pleasure with the Divine realm by inviting God to the party, the orgasmic pleasure is more potent, the connection to Source is magnified, and creative energy is empowered. It is our Divine Design.

Many people experience a disconnect between their relationship with God and sex. Do you? One reason for this is that we were sexually repressed for thousands of years through societal and religious standards, making it out to be the ultimate sin, compartmentalizing sex in one box and God in another. This disconnect also exists because God Source is often perceived as the Father, or Mother/Father God. We don't want to invite our parents into the bedroom; that's just weird.

The essence of God Source is in all relationships, mother, father, and also that of sister, brother, child, friend, and the lover. With this awareness, you can open yourself to integrate your sexual expression with your connection to the lover essence of God Source. Integrating your sexual pleasure with your connection to God is the core essence of a Sacred Sexuality practice.

Invite the lover essence of God Source into your sexual orgasmic experience, for the purpose of sharing its beauty. You can do this without breath activation and still feel a beautiful connection. After all, you're always breathing whether shallow or activated. However, the difference is similar to that between the mist setting on a garden hose compared to the jet stream setting. With the breath intentionally activated to channel your orgasmic energy through your nervous system and beyond your body, the connection is more focused and intensified.

AIR AND BREATH

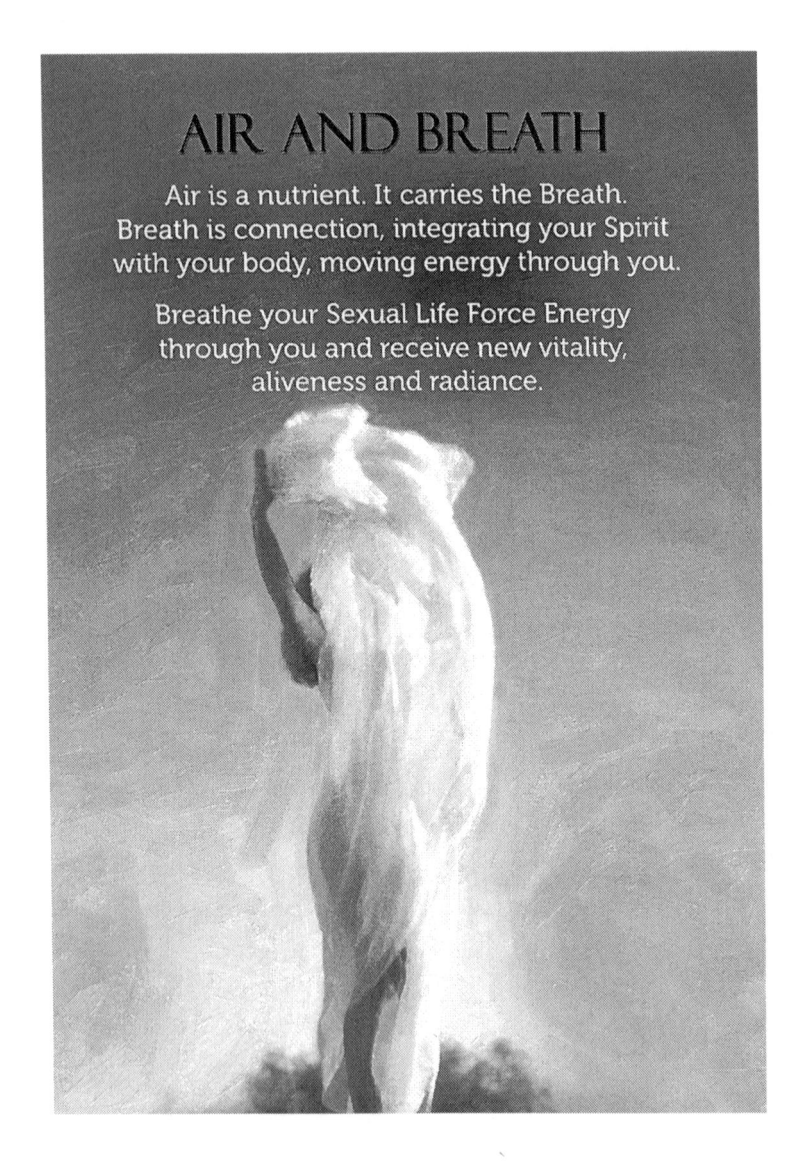

Air is a nutrient. It carries the Breath.
Breath is connection, integrating your Spirit
with your body, moving energy through you.

Breathe your Sexual Life Force Energy
through you and receive new vitality,
aliveness and radiance.

MIRACULOUS CYCLE & BRILLIANCE OF BREATH

Our bodies are miracles of creation. The catch is, we don't come with a manual. There are so many powerful ways to work with our breath and our sexual life force energy. When we combine this with the Invitation, what we experience is truly magical. The more we explore, learn and practice, the more we experience the extraordinary power of our Divine Design.

The presence of our breath in our body, is the presence of our essence in our body. If you've ever been with someone making their transition at their time of death, then you know you can feel their spirit separate from the body as they breathe their last breath. The heart and other organs are still shutting down, but their spirit... their essence leaves the body with that last breath.

Since Atma is essence/breath/soul, you can understand how consciously activating your breath to move and channel energy through your body can be so potent. The breath is not just a bunch of air going in and out of you. It is your very essence, your spirit.

The heart and lungs are the only two organs physically connected together. No wonder the breath is so powerful for healing the wounds of the heart.

The breath works in synch with our spinal cord and the peripheral nervous system. We can consciously direct our sexual orgasmic energy to move beyond the genital area and up throughout the entire body by tapping into the power of our breath.

When we activate the power of our breath in this way with our heart open, extending Invitation to Source, our orgasmic pleasure and our connection to Source expands. It's how we're designed or this would not be possible. A magical cycle happens through this connection of our physical nervous system, breath, heart, sexual energy and our Invitation to Divine Source.

During conception, we are transported from the Spirit realm through the act of sex which integrates us into our physical body. The first part of us that develops in the womb is the heart. The rest of the body develops around the heart. Once outside the womb, our first breath gives us life in our physical body.

"If you cannot face directly into your Sexuality, you will never discover your true Spirituality. Your Earthly Spirit leads to discovering your Heavenly Spirit.

Look at what created you to discover what will immortalize (heal) you."

~ *Hsi Lai; White Tigress Manual*

We have the ability to integrate our physical nervous system with our breath to amplify our energy. When our heart is open, connected to love as we breathe the orgasmic energy up our body, we can experience a merging with the Divine transcendental realm in a very tangible way.

THE CYCLE

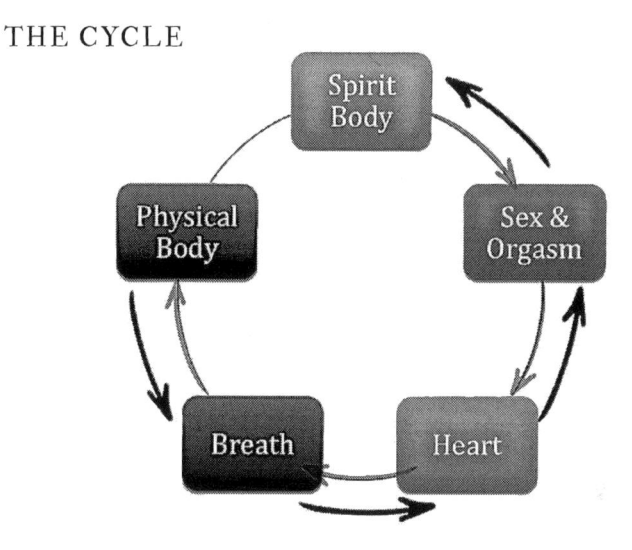

Diagram: A circular cycle with five nodes connected by arrows going both clockwise and counter-clockwise: Spirit Body → Sex & Orgasm → Heart → Breath → Physical Body → Spirit Body.

In this diagram, the arrows going clockwise show the cycle of merging the spirit body with the physical body. The counter clockwise arrows show the cycle of merging the physical body with the spirit body.

Sexual energy is powerful and potent. When you have sex, you are opening a vortex. When sex is activated with a closed heart or abusive, it can open a vortex of darkness into your energy field. When sex is heart connected and infused with love, the experience is joyful and you open a vortex to the Divine.

Sex plants the seed that creates the development of the heart in the womb. The heart opens us to the Sacred Sexual experience. The breath gives us physical life and it and moves our sexual life force energy through us. The breath empowers *The Invitation* as we merge with the Divine transcendental realm. This is the miraculous cycle and the brilliance of breath.

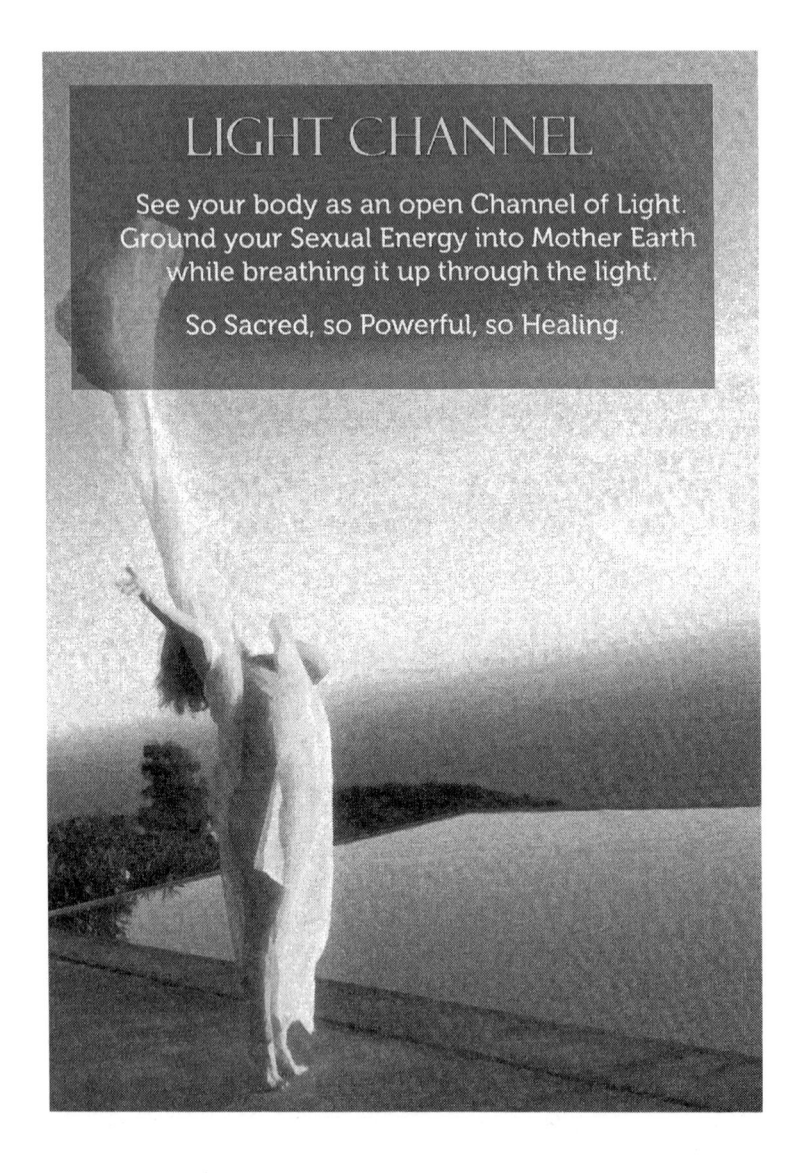

190 THE FOUR SACRED LAWS OF SEXUAL ENLIGHTENMENT

LIGHT CHANNEL

See your body as an open Channel of Light.
Ground your Sexual Energy into Mother Earth
while breathing it up through the light.

So Sacred, so Powerful, so Healing.

LIGHT CHANNEL

We are multi-dimensional beings. We are both matter and energy. While our physical body lives on Planet Earth, the part of us that is Spirit, that is Atma, exists within our physical body and the transcendental realm simultaneously. Our Spirit is not limited to our physical body. It is pure energy, love intelligence. It cannot be confined within matter. It merges with it.

Our bodies are light channels, a conduit between the physical realm and the nonphysical realm. Creating a deep connection with Source energy can be euphoric. It's no wonder so many of us spend so much time seeking this connection while here in a physical body.

Once you've had a taste of this euphoria and have touched the truth of your Divinity, there is no turning back. The Divine realm is, after all, where we come from. It is home. It is more natural to us than the density of the physical realm. We inhabit our physical bodies for a brief moment in time. We are visitors here.

"The subject of Sexuality is not in and of itself Spirituality, but Sexuality combined with your connection to who you are (a Divine Being), now that's an Orgasm!"

~ Abraham-Hicks; nonphysical intelligence channeled by Esther Hicks

---

WE CAME to this physical realm because wanted the physical experience. We wanted to experience and connect with the joy that our body and this magnificent planet has to offer. We wanted to experience the expansion we can create here. We wanted to share our touch and our love with others in the physical body.

Our root chakra is called the root for a reason. It connects us, roots us, and grounds us to the Earth, anchoring us to the physical realm. This is especially important to remember when practicing the Invitation with your sexual energy.

When you activate your breath to move orgasmic energy up your body and out your crown, it can leave you feeling scattered. The energy must be grounded. As you breathe the energy up your spine, at the same time focus on anchoring the orgasm into the Earth, so as you experience the euphoria you stay grounded in your body.

The self-pleasure practice of the Invitation is beautiful and multidimensional. Sharing with a partner in Divine Union magnifies the energy even more, creating the sweetest and most pleasurable of symphonies.

DIVINE UNION
"Divine Union with Spirit and Primal Expression
on Earth creates peace and ecstasy within.
With flesh intertwined, breathe in the Divine,
looking deep in the eyes of your Beloved.
Heart to heart, breath to breath, soul to soul."
~ Sacred Sexual Enlightenment Wisdom Cards

SELF-PLEASURE

In Chapter five, *The Gift*, I shared how the practice of self-pleasure can be fulfilling on all levels... physically, emotionally and spiritually. The Invitation is your secret ingredient to create the beauty of multidimensional self-pleasure. The Invitation as a solo practice takes masturbation beyond the physical and raises it to a high vibrational soul and heart opening experience. It merges your orgasmic energy and the love within you, with the love of the Divine realm.

The purpose of a self-pleasure ceremony is not to replace a lover unless your desire is to remain solo. Rather it contributes to feeling complete with your love of self. This way you do not go looking for your person from a place of neediness or to fill a void, you attract someone because they reflect your love, because it is a joy to be in one another's presence and to bear witness to one another's life.

"When you are the love of your life, then you meet someone who is also the love of their life and together it is a dream of unconditional love." ~ *Don Jose Ruiz*

If it brings you joy to have sexual fantasies about a real-life person, have fun with that. As you invite the lover essence of God Source to join you in your self-pleasure, you can give them any face, body, skin color, voice or gender you want, including that of someone you know. Just don't be attached to that person you know actually becoming your lover in real life, as we cannot manipulate the reality of another.

> *BELOVED'S PRESENCE*
> *"To call in a Beloved, invite the Lover Essence*
> *of the Divine into a Self-love Ceremony.*
> *Imagine your hands are your Beloved's hands,*
> *touching you how you desire to be touched.*
> *Feel their Essence loving you.*
> *Imagine their Presence Being with you."*
> *~ Sacred Sexual Enlightenment Wisdom Cards*

When I offer the Invitation during self-pleasure and tune into the lover essence of Source, I say something like, "My beautiful Divine lover, come and experience my love, my beautiful body and this pleasure with me."

In the self-pleasure Invitation, I feel a different presence enter my space from that of my Divine Team who joins me in meditation, healing sessions and as my guides. They feel more like a mother, father, mentor or sibling presence. The presence that joins me in my self-pleasure Invitation embodies the lover energy.

Perhaps he carries the essence of a lover whom I've experienced in another life. Perhaps he is the essence of a lover I have yet to experience in this life. This is my experience. It may not be yours. It's a personal practice. Notice what shows up for you. As long as you infuse it with love, it will be beautiful.

In 2011, I rented a condo in a gated community in Palm Springs. My condo was right next to the swimming pool and Jacuzzi. One night I was working on my computer through the night. At around 4:00 am, I went outside to have a hot soak in the Jacuzzi before heading to bed. Usually, the jets in the Jacuzzi did not work at night, but on this night, they were running full force.

With all my neighbors asleep, I had complete privacy. I removed my bathing suit to enjoy the water in the nude. As you may be aware, it is easy for a woman to bring herself to orgasm with the force of a Jacuzzi jet against her body. That's exactly what I did. I created a sacred self-pleasure ceremony with the help of the Jacuzzi.

I stood in front of a water jet activating my orgasmic energy. I channeled the energy through my breath, anchoring the orgasm down through my root chakra and into the Earth. At the same time, I breathed the energy up my spine, and out my crown chakra, while inviting my Divine lover to share in the beauty of my pleasure. As the climax of my orgasm erupted, I raised my hands and held them up to the sky. I spoke out loud and said, "I have to teach this to other women!"

In that exact moment, I saw a large bird in the distance flying toward me in the night sky. At first, I thought it may be a hawk. My immediate thought was, "What is a bird of prey doing out at night?"

As the bird flew closer, my orgasmic energy was still flowing. The bird flew directly over me through the exact center point where my arms were outstretched sharing my pleasure with Spirit. When the bird was over my head, I could clearly see it was a Snowy White Owl. I gasped in awe and delight.

When I left the Jacuzzi, I went into the house and opened my *Animal Speak* book by Ted Andrews to see what message White Owl had brought me. There it was… White Owl represents feminine wisdom. It reminds us of the secrets we keep as it flies at night. It also teaches there is strength in gentleness. How perfect that this messenger of feminine wisdom flew directly over me in my orgasmic moment; so magical.

At the time, I only worked with women, so those were the words spoken during my ceremony. However, this Sacred Sexual practice of the Invitation is equally powerful for men. The message White Owl brings, is for the feminine within each of us. So, beautiful men, this also applies to you.

ENERGY ATTRACTION

Everything in the Universe is energy, including us. Energy cannot be created and it cannot be destroyed. Energy attracts like energy. Sexual energy is powerful and potent in its frequency, so it is especially important that you are infusing this frequency with a positive flow of pure love.

Be impeccable with your energy. Whatever energy you are emanating is the energy you will attract more of to you. Do what you need to do to make sure your energy is clear and of a positive frequency. Is there anyone left to forgive? Are you being responsible? Are you honoring the gift of yourself and the person you are sharing yourself with? Life is sexually transmitted. What are you infusing it with? Infuse it with love.

We live in a Universe of free will. Assumptions are not made on your behalf. You are Creator. The Universe is serving you, taking your lead. When you have sex, you open an energy vortex. If you are not impeccable with your energy and you have sex while angry or distracted by frustrations at work, you are attracting energy beings that are of the same frequency into your vortex. Be impeccable with your energy. When you have sex and that vortex opens, what are you letting in? You get to make that choice.

Moments of anger in relationships happen. If this happens consistently in your relationship, then you may want to abstain from sex until you have done what you need to do to come to a place of resolve and peace with one another.

If your relationship is mostly in harmony and you're simply having a tense moment, having sex can be a beautiful way to release the tension. Before diving in, take a moment to see past the tension as you gaze into one another's eyes. Command that everything released is carried into the light to be used for other means. Visualize your tension being transmuted into the light. Connect with the love and divinity within your lover and within yourself. Then release your tension through sex from this space.

Before a client arrives in my studio, I take time to energetically prepare the space. I extend the Invitation before my client arrives, asking permission for their Divine Team to work with my Divine Team, guiding me to be there for them in the highest way to provide the most beautiful deepest healing experience possible.

During the breath work sessions, my clients release a lot of sadness, anger, and rage. I command that all energy released goes into the light to be used for other means. If I did not do this, the heaviness of the sadness, anger, and rage would remain in my space. After every session, I literally take out the energetic garbage with the help of my Divine Team.

Burning sage, spraying essential oils and sound toning are all good for cleansing the energy in your space. I love to invite Divine light to fill every fragment of my home. Sometimes I play beautiful uplifting music and dance in the space to infuse it with my love, while extending the Invitation to my Divine Team to feel the joy in my body and join in the dance with me. I give impeccable attention to the energy of my home and my healing space. How do you care for the energy of the environment in your home and your body?

Sexual energy is powerful enough to create a new human being. When activated, it is like blasting out an energetic broadcast with an enormous high-powered frequency. When you host a party at your home, you are discerning with whom you invite. You want only those of a positive frequency in your home. Take the same care and discernment with your energy when having sex. Choose your partners and timing wisely. Only allow the love and joy of the Divine within you be the energy you emanate and attract.

SACRED CEREMONY

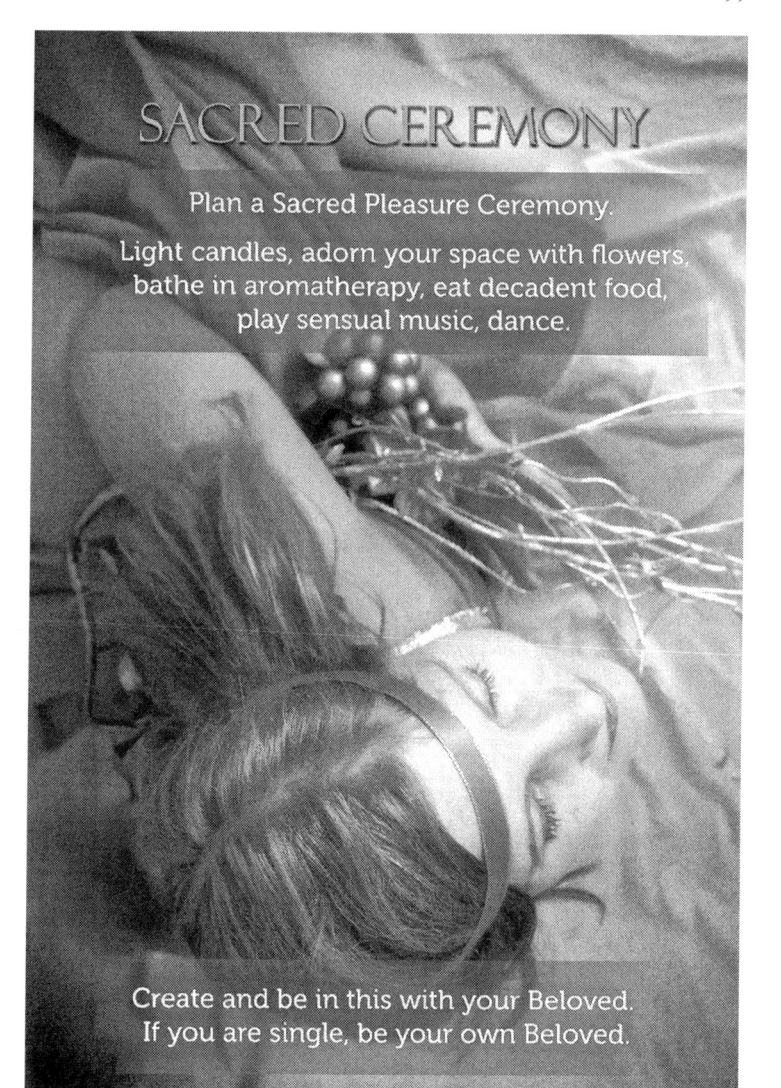

Plan a Sacred Pleasure Ceremony.

Light candles, adorn your space with flowers, bathe in aromatherapy, eat decadent food, play sensual music, dance.

Create and be in this with your Beloved.
If you are single, be your own Beloved.

THE INVITATION CEREMONY

The following is a suggestion for how you can create your own Invitation ceremony as a couple. If you are solo, improvise to make it work for you. The process is mostly the same.

You will be gazing deeply into the left eye of your lover throughout this process. This is not like staring at one another. It is a soft gentle gaze. Sometimes you may break your gaze and close your eyes as you bask in the pleasure of the experience. Just remember to bring your awareness back to eye contact.

We see deeper into the soul of another through the left eye. If you're skeptical, try gazing into the left eye, then switch to the right eye. You will notice the difference. It's just the way our brains are wired.

The Invitation ceremony can be done in the spur of the moment. All you need is an open heart, pure intention and the desire to extend the Invitation to Source. It is also especially beautiful when you plan it in advance. The following are some suggestions to make that happen…

1. PREPARATION:

Write down everything that you want to have present during your Invitation ceremony. Imagine the most beautiful experience you can. What do you see? What do you hear? What do you smell? What do you touch? What do you taste? Then make a list. Gather up all the things on the list you have already have and purchase the rest. The following are some suggestions:

- Your favorite flowers
- Fragrance for your bath
- Massage oil (pure organic coconut oil is best for genitals)
- A special bowl for the oil"
- A hot plate to heat the oil
- Extra soft sheets
- Extra soft towels
- Candles
- Incense, sage or aromatherapy oils
- Lingerie
- Chocolate
- Fresh fruit
- Create a special playlist of music

Schedule uninterrupted time for your ceremony. Prepare the space with the details from your list and make your space beautiful and sensual. You can create this together, or one of you can create it as a surprise for the other. Imagine how delicious it will be to adorn your space and have it prepared with music playing, candles burning and delicious fruit to eat. Then surprise your lover with a note, inviting them to come join you as you wait for them wearing beautiful lingerie, a sarong or fully in the nude.

Do the preparation in silence or play uplifting soothing music; chant or sing a favorite song. Give your full attention to the intention you are creating. You can begin your Invitation during the preparation. Speak to the lover essence of Source. Say a prayer to Divine Source and communicate what you are intending and preparing for, inviting God Source Energy Love to share in the beauty with you.

Maybe you want to dance around the room in celebration of your beautiful bodies and souls coming together. Dance is a high vibration activity. When we play uplifting heart centered music and dance, we infuse the space with our light and our love. Be creative. Infuse the space with sensuality and with your precious love.

REFLECTION
"Gaze into the left eye of your
Beloved and synchronize your breath.
Relax your bodies.
Breathe deeply and slowly.
Really FEEL them. SEE the Divine in them.
Savor the Reflection of You through them
and allow it to take you to bliss."
~ Sacred Sexual Enlightenment Wisdom Cards

2. THE CEREMONY:

Once your space is set up, sit in stillness and connect deeply to your breath as you softly gaze into one another's eyes. Tune into the sound of the breath moving in and out of your bodies. Tune into the love within your hearts.

Then, when you are ready, begin with touch. Start by placing your hands over one another's heart. If you are solo, connect with your heart space first then touch your body. Touch one another slowly in awe and wonderment, exploring your bodies as if it is your first time. Notice the texture of the skin, the contours of curves, the strength of muscles, and your sensitivity to this touch. See the body as the beautiful miracle it is. Breathe in your own beauty and the beauty of your lover.

See the beauty of the light in your lover's eyes, gazing into them steady and deep. If you are solo, look into a mirror so you can see the light of love in your own eyes. After all, you are the love of your life. Now extend The Invitation again. As you see the Divine reflected back to you through your lover's eyes, give thanks for this presence of Divine love in your sacred space.

Now, make love, have sex. Slowly savor each other and the bliss of every moment. If you are solo, make love to yourself. Breathe deeply into your orgasmic energy, extending it and expanding it for as long as you can. Synchronize your breath. Breathe your orgasmic energy up your spinal column, nourishing all of your body with your orgasm. Then as your orgasm becomes climatic, send it down into the Earth to ground it, while also channeling it through your breath up and out of your bodies merging with the Divine realm. Feel how beautiful it is sharing your orgasmic energy with Source in this way.

When grounding your energy with a partner, visualize it going through your lover's body and down through their root chakra. Make eye contact with them as you do this, and they will feel greater depth of connection.

Once the peak of the orgasmic release subsides, stay with the orgasm. It's not over yet. Place your hands on one another's heart. If you are solo, place your hands over your own heart. Continue to stay fully present with the ripple of energy still moving through your bodies. Feel it in your fingers, your face, your chest and down to your toes. Feel the presence of God Source love around you and within you. Bask in the beauty of the experience you just created.

THE ART OF ORGASMIC CREATION

"The desire for sexual expression is by far the strongest and most impelling of all the human emotions, and for this very reason this desire, when harnessed and transmuted into action, other than that of physical expression, may raise one to the status of a genius." ~ *Napoleon Hill*

BECAUSE SEXUAL ORGASM is powerful enough to create a human life, it makes sense that it is powerful enough to fuel all that we wish to create. Skeptics may argue that creating a human is not about energy flow, rather a simple biological fact of the egg and the sperm working together. I say it is both. The energy of the orgasm has to build until it comes to a climactic explosion strong enough to release the sperm. Although a woman can be impregnated without her orgasmic energy building, we cannot deny the incredible power of orgasmic energy.

You are a magnificent manifestor, an artist. You are always creating your reality, whether it's one you want or not. You are pure love, pure energy, life and vibration.

Everything in this physical reality began with a thought. The focus of thought, the vibration behind it and the action taken, brings it into reality. Orgasmic energy plugged into God Source love greatly enhances your vibrational field.

When giving focus to what you want to create, notice what is uncomfortable about it. For example, if you want to attract your person, but you fear you will never meet them and grow old alone, allow yourself to feel that fear. What are the thoughts around that, what are your feelings and your body sensations? Now that you've acknowledged it, it's not suppressed. Now by shifting into the beauty of attracting your person, the positive frequency of these feelings can neutralize the fear and doubt.

So, shift into the beauty of having your person in your life. Imagine they're already here. What do you see? What are your thoughts? Connect with the joyful feelings of having your beloved in your life. What body sensations come with that? Completely go into this beautiful vision and experience it as your own little virtual reality. You only need to stay there for about twenty seconds. Trust that within this time, the Universe received your message. The seed has been planted. If you still feel doubt, acknowledge it. Then, shift back to the joy of your vision being a reality and connect with the joyful feelings and body sensations of that.

As I shared in *The Gift*, our creative life force energy and our sexual energy are one and the same, both activated within the Sacral Chakra area. Orgasmic energy created you. You are an Orgasmic Creation. Combining the focused energy of your orgasm and breath with the focus of your vision increases the force behind your creation.

Here is an example of one of my personal Orgasmic

Creations: I was envisioning what my nonphysical Divine lover looked like, what his voice sounded like, how he made love to me, his smile, his height, his eye contact, his skin color. I communicated to Source I desired such a lover in the flesh and eventually, that is exactly what I received.

I was so specific with what I wanted and had such joy playing with my vision that a man who fit the exact same description walked into my home for a consultation. He was so in alignment with my vision he took my breath away. I discovered that his desire for me was equal. So, he never became a client. We chose to be lovers instead.

What a powerful Orgasmic Creation. I didn't go looking. He just walked into my home. I was also clear at that time that although I wanted a lover, I did not have time for a relationship. So, I manifested a lover with a very busy schedule who did not want a relationship either. We had few opportunities to connect, but when we did it was beautiful. So just remember specificity plays an important role. Be careful what you ask for.

I will share with you a simple practice you can do to empower your manifestation abilities with your orgasmic energy. If you are doing this with a partner, I recommend you both focus on the same vision simultaneously. There is power in numbers when you have laser focus pointing in one direction. Get clear on what you both desire. It could be a new home, a vacation, a new car, a new business, a child, etc. This is your dream, your art. Create it.

If you believe what you want is money, you may want to take a closer look at your intention for manifestation. For fifteen years I worked for a large seminar company on their main stage as one of their lead facilitators. There were between 100 to 400 participants at each event, so I have guided thousands through this experience. The name of my process was called *Intention*.

The participants would write an intention they wanted to manifest on a piece of paper attached to a torch. (In my thirties and forties, I worked as a professional magician and I got really good at fire eating.) I would then teach the participants how to eat fire as a method of learning to move through their fears from a space of calm, while focused on their intention. Almost every time, when someone struggled to put out the flame, it was because their intention was out of alignment. Most of the time, they had set their intention to make a specific amount of money in a specific amount of time.

I remember one example clearly. A woman could not get the flame out no matter how hard she tried. The flame burned for so long that the fuel was gone and it was just a small piece of burning cotton, as easy to blow out as a candle, yet she could not blow it out.

When I asked her what her intention was, tears streamed down her face and she said, "To manifest two million dollars in two years."

I asked, "What do you want two million dollars for?"

She said, "To spend more time with my daughter and to open a new school."

I said, "That's your intention, not the two million dollars. The money is just one of the possibilities of how your intention can happen. The *how* is not your job. You don't know how it will happen. You may meet a business partner who wants to invest. Change your intention to wanting to spend more time with your daughter and open a new school."

She did. She lit the torch again and got it out first try.

In all the years I've facilitated this process I've seen this scenario play itself out repeatedly. The participants get stuck on the *how* verses their true intention and they can't move forward. Once they align with their true intention, their mind is clear, their energy opens up and their body relaxes.

When you plant a seed, you fill the pot with soil, you water it and give it sunshine. You trust the seed is planted, nourished and will grow. If you keep digging up the soil to see if the seed is growing, you prevent its growth.

The same is true for any manifestation practice. You need not ask for the same thing over and over again. That's like digging up the seed. It infuses your vision with doubt, interfering with its creation. Plant the seed, nourish it with the light of your love and the love of Source, and then trust. After the Invitation ceremony, stay in the joy of your intention and take inspired action.

When you combine clarity of vision, strength of faith, joy in your body, aligned with the love of Source and surrender to the *how*, you open to a flow of possibility. The Universe is magical in how it can surprise you beyond your imagination. Imagine the turbo charge when you fuel this with pure intentions and your orgasmic life force energy.

As you do the Orgasmic Creation Ceremony, honor your sexual energy as *The Gift*. Enter this practice in a space of peacefulness and Forgiveness with everyone from your past so your energy is calm, clear and infused with light.

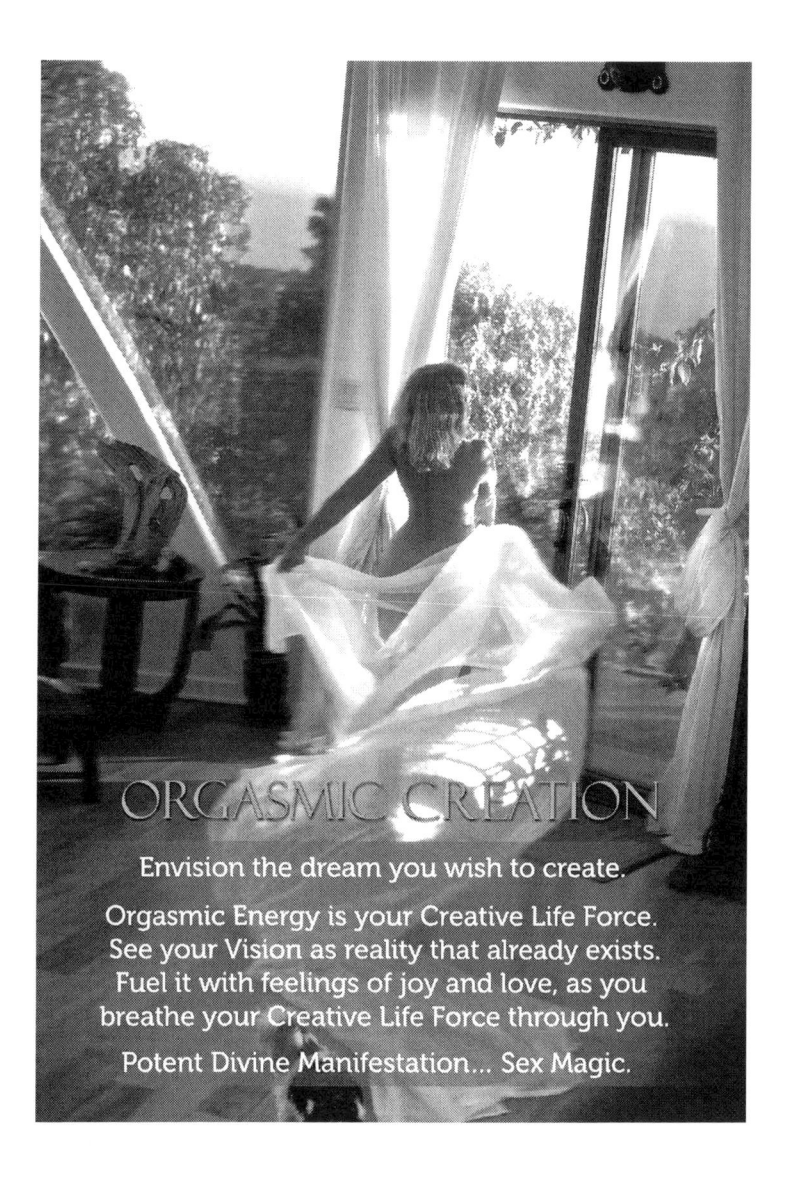

ORGASMIC CREATION

Envision the dream you wish to create.

Orgasmic Energy is your Creative Life Force.
See your Vision as reality that already exists.
Fuel it with feelings of joy and love, as you
breathe your Creative Life Force through you.

Potent Divine Manifestation... Sex Magic.

ORGASMIC CREATION CEREMONY

In my online program, we explore in great depth, all the layers of The Four Sacred Laws of Sexual Enlightenment, including how to fully activate the power of Orgasmic Creation. This includes breath work, guided meditations, mentorship, experiential processes and private sessions for individual attention. It's always more powerful to work together through live video and in person, but for this book, I will share the best I can on how to create an Orgasmic Creation Ceremony.

This Ceremony is basically the same whether solo or with a partner. Choose one vision at a time to give your focus to. If you are with a partner, be in agreement of what that vision is before you begin. Then proceed.

1. ENVIRONMENT:

Prepare your environment first. Begin by finding an image that represents what you want to create in your life. If you paint, even better. Create your own image. Put the image up where you have a good visual of it. Whenever you look at it, feel the joy of it.

For this ceremony, choose a space in your home that feels most like a sanctuary. Make sure it is clean and clear of clutter. Remove any distractions. Adjust the lighting so it feels beautiful to you, whether that is the lighting of candles or letting the warmth of the sunlight shine through a window. Create a beautiful sensual environment the same as I described in the Invitation Ritual.

2. STILLNESS:

Being in stillness may bring more detail into your vision. Receive it. Allow the information to flow through.

Sit comfortably. If you are doing this in partnership, sit facing one another. Start by softly gazing into one another's eyes, fully connect with your love of self and of one another. If solo, place your hands over your heart and feel the love within you.

Now close your eyes and place all of your focus on your breath. Take deep relaxing breaths in through your nose, exhaling out through your mouth. Bring all your attention to the sound of the breath moving in and out of your body. Feel every part of your body relax more and more with each exhalation.

If you find your mind wandering, bring your attention back to the sound of your breath moving through your body. Notice how your breath enters your body as cool air going in, warming inside, warm breath out. As you focus on your breath in this way, the busyness in the mind will calm.

3. FOCUS:

Surrender to the stillness. With your attention on the breath, bring the vision of your intention into your thoughts. Glance at the image of your vision whenever you need help with focus. Then bring your attention back to your mind's eye and imagination. See your vision in your mind as though it already exists. Feel the joy that comes with having this thing in your life.

If you are doing this with your lover, speak out loud and share the thoughts flowing through you. Share what you see and how beautiful it makes you feel. What body sensations do you have? In your mind's eye, continue to see your vision blossom. Stay with the joy of it. See it and feel it as if it is already a reality.

If your vision is a professional one, be sure to give attention to how your vision is of benefit to others and the joy it brings them.

4. INVITATION AND SUPPORT:

From this space of joy and focus, invite God Source into your experience to share in the joy of the pleasure you are activating and the beauty of your vision.

Now you will add a layer and request support. Give thanks to your Divine Team for orchestrating what needs to happen for your vision to blossom into reality.

Asking your Divine Team can be powerful in receiving support with the manifestation process. A great way to start a question commonly used in the Access Consciousness practices is, "What would it take _____?"

For example, "What would it take for me to meet my ideal person to share my love and life with?"

Or, "What would it take for me to receive five new ideal clients whose lives will be transformed by my work?"

When you ask a question in this way, without attachment, their role is to answer. This can show up as inspiration to take a specific action. For example, a week later, you may feel a strong impulse to shop at the new grocery store on your way home and you meet the love of your life. Trust and have faith it is done. Your job is to surrender and let go of the need to know how, stay open to the possibilities, and take inspired action.

Now that you have invited Source Energy into this ceremony, you are ready to build your energy and infuse your vision with your potent sexual life force energy.

5. ORGASMIC CHARGE:

Stay with the beauty of your vision, the joy of it, your love of self, one another and Source. Aligned with the purity of your love, activate your orgasmic energy.

As you build your orgasmic energy, activate your breath to move and channel the orgasmic energy throughout your body. Imagine that your inhale begins at your root chakra and draw your orgasmic energy up your spine with your breath, all the way to your brain and your third eye where you hold the vision. While doing this, also feel your root grounded into the Earth, and the presence of Divine love with you.

On the exhale, relax the energy back down the front of your body. Continue to do this circular breath motion as you become more and more aroused. Contracting your PC muscle on the inhale and relaxing it on the exhale can help you with this.

If you find it challenging to stay focused on your vision, activate your breath, and raise your orgasmic energy all at the same time, then breathe normally at first. If your mind wanders away from your vision, glance at the print or painting of it to bring it back into focus. Notice if your shoulders are becoming tense or engaged. If so, relax them using the exhale to help you. The only part of your body that you want engaged is your breath, your PC muscle, and your orgasmic energy. As the orgasmic energy builds and becomes stronger, trust the seed of your vision is now planted.

As you feel your orgasmic energy building, surrender to it, versus trying to make it happen. It's common for the body to contract when orgasmic energy builds. Notice if that happens and use your breath to fully relax and surrender to it. Surrender to the pleasure. Surrender the need to reach the goal of climax.

If you are doing this with your lover be patient with yourselves as you discover the flow. You may discover it works best to self-pleasure yourselves first. If you choose to do this, while self-pleasuring, make eye contact and stay connected to your heart and with each other. Once your orgasmic energy has built up, join in yab yum. Yab yum is when you have intercourse while sitting upright with the woman on the lap of the man, so you can maintain eye contact and a heart to heart connection. If yab yum is uncomfortable for you to do on a bed or on the floor, try using a chair, or choose another position. This is your ceremony. Explore it.

As you feel the orgasmic energy getting ready to peak, hold your vision in your mind or glance at the photo or painting. Do not climax yet. Hold it back. Use your breath and squeeze your PC muscles to help you. Take your orgasm to the edge and then pull it back, then build it back up again. Do this a few times before releasing the orgasm. Stay connected. Be playful. Have fun with it.

Ride the wave as much as possible without ejaculation or

climatic release. You can even keep the climax of your orgasm inside your body. If so, I recommend you do this as a morning practice, so as you go about your day, you have this beautiful buildup of sexual creative life force energy you can channel into inspired action.

If you choose to release the orgasmic climax, it's beautiful to do this practice near the end of the day, so as you drift off to sleep, you take the power of the energy and your vision into your dream state. Either way, morning afternoon or evening, it's all good.

If you choose to climax, as you feel your orgasm peaking, open your eyes and make eye contact with your lover. See your vision and their love reflected back to you as this potent creative life force energy surges through you. It's beautiful if you climax simultaneously, but not imperative to the process. As the orgasmic energy releases ground it down through your root, while at the same time you draw it up with your breath, through your body, to your third eye.

Savor the ripples and after waves of the orgasmic energy moving through you. As your energy subsides, relax your breath. Maintain eye contact, staying fully tuned into every sensation down to your fingers and toes. Press down on one another's thighs with a massaging motion to help ground each other. If you are going solo, massage your own thighs.

If you have trees outside your window, look at them and breathe their beauty into your body. Complete by placing your hands over one another's heart. If you are solo, place your hands over your own your heart. Feel the connection to your love and to Source.

Once you feel your energy anchored, take a moment to notice what came up for you. Did the vision take on more detail? Did it get stronger, did it fade? Did it shift in a way you did not expect? If so, how do you feel about that? Share the answers to these questions with your partner and anything else that comes up for you. You may want to journal about your experience, especially if you are doing the process solo.

Most of all, stay in the beauty of the energy you just created. Continue to infuse this practice with your love… your love for you, your love for your partner and your love for God Source. Surrender and be in the joy of this love.

SUMMARY

Once you get used to including the Invitation in your sexual experience, you will want to do so regularly. At times only indulging in pure raw primal sex may be your choice. There is no judgment or right or wrong way here. Source energy has no expectations. You are Creator. You get to decide how you activate your own energy and body.

The Four Sacred Laws in this book are in the order they are for a reason. By implementing the first three Laws, the Invitation feels even sweeter and more potent. I like to think of the Invitation as the icing on the cake.

Sharing your love with Source is always sweet and beautiful. When you integrate and embody the first three Sacred Laws, the Invitation is free of hesitation or emotional residue, allowing you to open more fully to the connection and magic of the Invitation experience. The result is a Sacred Sexuality practice embodied with inner peacefulness, joy and Awakened Ecstasy.

Embrace your sexual energy as the Gift it is. Take care of your emotional well-being and be in Forgiveness with everyone, especially yourself. Be in alignment and in integrity. Take full Responsibility for your words, actions and creation, free from ego, always heart centered.

The more you practice the Invitation, merging your love and orgasmic flow with the Divine realm, the more magic you experience. You may even have out of body experiences.

Savor the deliciousness of you, the expansion of your love... your love of self, Spirit and one another, and your potent orgasmic sexual life force energy. Bask in the beauty of your Divine Design in all its glory and magnificence.

APPLYING THE 4TH SACRED LAW TO THE WORKPLACE

Infuse your sexual life force energy with your love and your joy. Infuse your sexual life force energy into the passion of your work. Extend the Invitation to your Divine Team to share in the beauty of this. Move forward and take action from this space with the intention to serve and be of benefit to others.

Social media has had a dramatic impact on marketing. The in your face type of promotion is outdated and a turn-off. The more your ideal clients feel the essence and integrity of your work and the passion behind it, the more they will be drawn to it.

Be aware of getting so caught up in the details of logistics that you lose the essence of what your work is about. The core essence of you is your love, joy and the passion that lives within your heart.

What is the big why behind your product, service or message? How does it serve and benefit others? Make that your priority. Connect with the essence of your work and from that space take your next action step.

"Sexual energy is the creative energy of virtually all geniuses. There never has been and never will be a great leader, builder or artist lacking in this driving force of sex." ~ *Napoleon Hill*

Summing It All Up

It's time for us to create a world where discussion and expression around sexuality is more evolved and awakened. It's time for us to live in a world where it is common practice to honor and savor the gift of it, the healing of it, the sacredness of it, the responsibility of it and how to create Spiritual alignment with it. It's time to create a new sexual legacy for the generations who follow.

Orgasmic energy resets your autonomic nervous system. It is the fountain of youth. It releases the love hormone of oxytocin and the feel good hormone serotonin. Orgasm makes your skin glow, it gives you more radiance, brighter eyes, and a more flexible and stimulated mind. When you embrace and integrate who you are as both a Sexual and Divine Being while implementing the *Four Sacred Laws of Sexual Enlightenment*, life on Earth is a delicious life giving, loving, co-creative ecstatic experience. This is your birthright. It's time to reclaim this, your Divine Design.

It is my intention that this book is a reminder of the beautiful creation of your Divine Design and for you to experience more of the joy and Awakened Ecstasy of that.

I will continue to embrace and embody a delicious God infused orgasmic existence. If you would like some help along the way, you know where to find me. The honor is mine.

Let's do this together.

Think of me as your Call Girl.

Because…

I call upon the light that I see in you to shine unapologetically in the world.

I call upon the inner child in you that is crying to come out and play.

I call upon the presence of peace that lives within your spirit body to be fully present in your physical sexual body.

I call upon the Creator in you to surrender to the calling in you that is hungry to be fulfilled.

Beloved, what are you willing to call upon?

Much love to you,
- Jaitara

SUMMING IT ALL UP 221

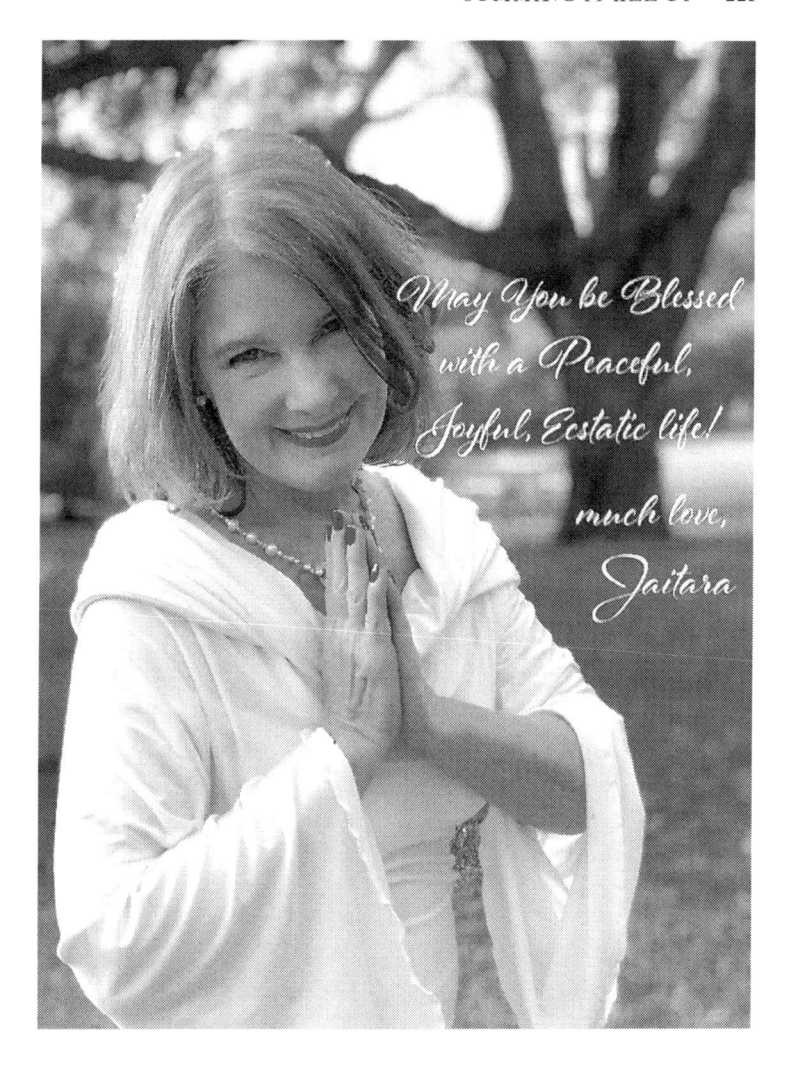

May You be Blessed with a Peaceful, Joyful, Ecstatic life!

much love,

Jaitara

TRIBUTE TO EVELINA

Evelina Pentcheva is a great blessing in my life. She is pure light, an inspiration and a forever soul mate sister friend.

This book and the *Sacred Sexual Enlightenment Wisdom Cards* deck exists because of her love, generosity and brilliance of artistry. She is responsible for the cover design and all of the beautiful images inside this book.

I have witnessed her blossom into an exquisite writer and brilliant source of wisdom. She embodies what this book is about more than anyone I know… a pure example of Divinity expressed in human form.

Thank you, Evelina, for the blessing and gift of you.

"Tantra is the shortest path to awakening to the divine nature of all…

If you are attracted to it guided by your quest for pleasure… know that it's a pleasure beyond what your concept of pleasure is…

> *it's an opening to life…*
> *it's a sacred tremor...*
> *a dissolution of everything into nothing and nothing into everything…*
> *It's the reverberating of the entire expression of creation, of God… within your Heart."*

~ Evelina Pentcheva; Artist, Transformaational Photographer, and founder of *The Tantra of Presence*
TheTantraOfPresence.com

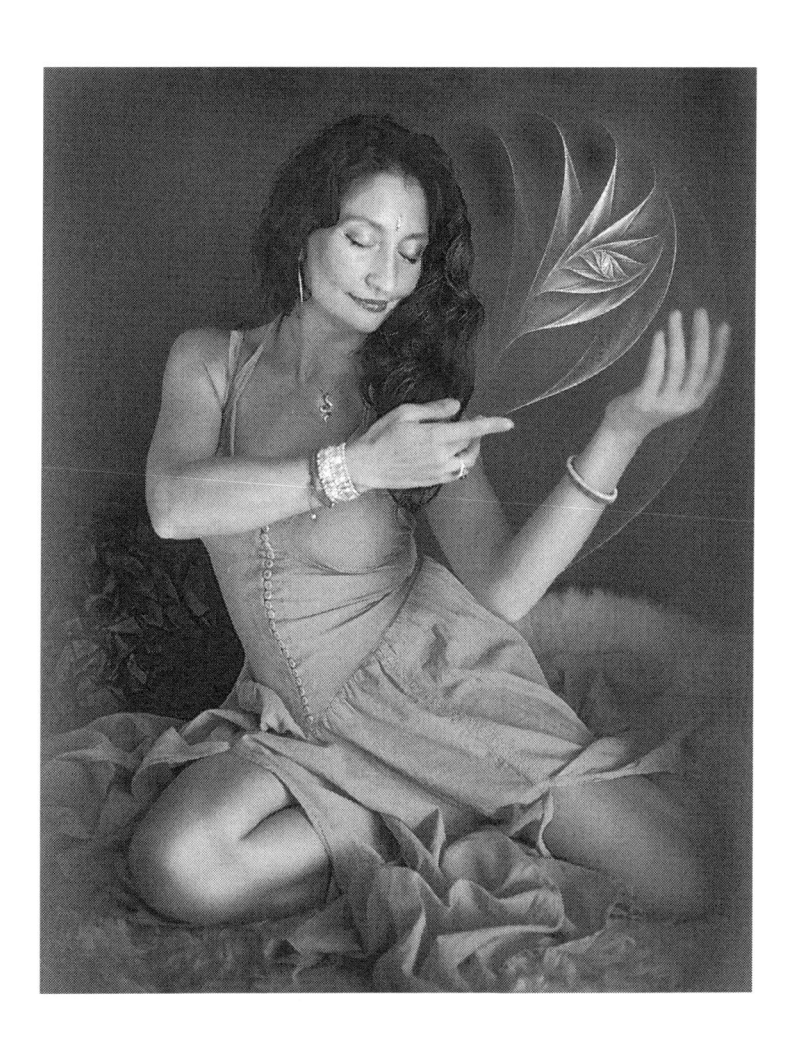

RESOURCES *and* OFFERINGS

The following are web addresses to support you to live a more joyful life, spiritually, emotionally, sexually and creatively. I look forward to connecting with you.
Much love,
Jaitara; Jaitara.com

Jaitara.com/Events — Details on online programs, live events, and women's retreats.

Jaitara.com/PrivateSessions — Healing, breath work, empowerment, intimacy and Tantric Sexuality coaching for couples and singles

Jaitara.com/Speaking — Details on speaking topics and training programs for corporations and events.

Jaitara.com/Store — Where you will find the following products, and more:
- *The Sacred Sexual Enlightenment Wisdom Cards*
- *Heal Your Sexual Legacy*™, the home study program, mentioned in Chapter 6
- *The Forgiveness Process*, free audio as shared in Chapter 6.

- *Discover Your Sacred Lover Body Types*™; free assessment and video
- Learn more about the PEMF Mats, mentioned in Chapter 7

DivineSagePublishing.com — Turn your brilliance into a best seller with our Awakened Author publishing programs. Offering full publishing services for Indie Authors, including book writing support, beautiful cover design and interior design, formatting, editing, marketing services, full administration set up for sale on Amazon and global distribution to book stores. We turn your book into a best seller and treat it the love it deserves.

EvelinaPentcheva.com — Evelina is my dear Sister friend and co-creative partner. She wrote the foreword, designed the book cover, is responsible for the photo art in this book and co-created the Sacred Sexual Enlightenment Wisdom Cards deck with me. Contact her to receive her photographic art services.

TheTantraOfPresence.com — Evelina Pentcheva is the founder and wisdom keeper of these beautiful uplifting and heart expanding events. She is an alchemist of inner connection, truth and transformation, working with groups or privately

MotivatingTheTeenSpirit.com — Communication with Youth, as shared in Chapter 7.

Made in the USA
Middletown, DE
06 May 2019